Basics in
Medical
Education

Basics in
Medical
Education

Zubair Amin
Khoo Hoon Eng

National University of Singapore

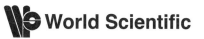

World Scientific

NEW JERSEY • LONDON • SINGAPORE • SHANGHAI • HONG KONG • TAIPEI • BANGALORE

Published by

World Scientific Publishing Co. Pte. Ltd.

5 Toh Tuck Link, Singapore 596224

USA office: 27 Warren Street, Suite 401-402, Hackensack, NJ 07601

UK office: 57 Shelton Street, Covent Garden, London WC2H 9HE

British Library Cataloguing-in-Publication Data
A catalogue record for this book is available from the British Library.

First published 2003
Reprinted 2006, 2007

BASICS IN MEDICAL EDUCATION

Royalties from the sale of this book will benefit basic health care needs of children in developing countries.

For photocopying of material in this volume, please pay a copying fee through the Copyright Clearance Center, Inc., 222 Rosewood Drive, Danvers, MA 01923, USA. In this case permission to photocopy is not required from the publisher.

ISBN-13 978-981-238-209-2
ISBN-10 981-238-209-7

Typeset by Stallion Press
Email: enquiries@stallionpress.com

Printed in Singapore by B & JO Enterprise

Foreword

Currently there is a vibrant and passionate debate on seemingly two contradictory positions of medical education establishments. One group muses on how successful the medical schools have been in recent years in cultivating society's best minds and transforming them into mature physicians. The other group's view is less congratulatory. The principal argument of this group is that medical schools are remarkably resistant to adopting the science of medical education. Medical schools are lagging far behind in the advancement in the science of education management. This group paints a gloomier future—either the medical establishment continues to adapt or face eventual atrophy. One may ponder how to reconcile these two seemingly opposing views. It may be that both viewpoints are true—medical schools *are* creating the best physicians but at the same time they are remarkably resistant to adopting new changes in learning and teaching paradigms.

Many argue, reasonably so, that there is a necessity to be cautious in adopting the fast-paced changes. The stakes are much higher and a false move is a move that we can ill- afford. Moreover, new is not synonymous with superiority. But, most believe there is a need to change—slow yet steady, cautious but determined at the same time.

Why are the medical faculty and medical schools so reluctant to change? One of the most important factors is the fear of the unknown—a substantial lack of knowledge about the science and art of teaching and learning in medicine. Ignorance breeds fear and fear perpetuates the collective inertia. The general lack of knowledge about teaching and learning among medical teachers is entirely understandable. Most medical teachers were taught in an era when the concepts of medical education were developing. Teaching was mostly teacher dominated, and there was very little emphasis on life-long and self-directed learning. Teaching was more of an art rather than a science without focus on empirical evidence to support the practice. But this cannot go on indefinitely.

Two of my colleagues and fellow medical education enthusiasts have completed the commendable task of bringing the teaching and learning concepts in medicine to the realm of general medical teachers. I am specifically delighted that the target reader of the book is medical teachers, as this is the segment within the medical establishment who needs the knowledge about medical education most. Throughout the book, they have maintained a delicate balance between the 'why' aspects of medical education emphasizing the needs for change and adaptation and the 'how' aspects demonstrating the way concepts and theories of medical education can be of immediate benefit to the medical teachers.

Teaching and learning is a much cherished activity; understanding the science behind teaching and learning should be an even more joyous and attractive pursuit. The book provides us with an easy yet essential reading to medical education. At the same time, it reminds us of the long journey that we eventually will be taking in keeping up our good job of producing efficient healers for society by gradually embracing what the rich and dynamic field of medical education has to offer.

Professor *Lee* Eng Hin
Dean, Faculty of Medicine
National University of Singapore
December 2002

Acknowledgements

The book is the collective efforts of ours over the last three years. Such an effort can only take place in the presence of supportive home and work environments and continued confidence of our friends and colleagues in our passions.

The support came in various ways: sustained encouragement, review and critique, providing flexibility at work and at home, and most of all, educating us on the many aspects of medical education.

Zubair Amin personally expresses his deep gratitude to his wife Sonia and their daughters Bushra and Samira, and to his parents Professor Aminul Haque and Mrs. Sitara Haque. Without their unconditional support, the book would not have materialized. He is also grateful to the following people for guiding and supporting his career: Drs. Leo G. Niederman, Georges Bordage, Ara Tekian, Robert Mrtek, Arthur Elstein, Mark Gelula, Wlodzimierz Wisniewski from the University of Illinois at Chicago (UIC); Drs. Tan Keng Wee, Lim Sok Bee, and Lawrence Chan from K K Women's and Children's Hospital; Drs. Rethy Chhem, Matthew Gwee and Koh Doh Rhoon from National University of Singapore, and Prof. M-Q K Talukder in Bangladesh.

Khoo Hoon Eng thanks Dr. Sharifah Hapsah Syed Baharuddin for first kindling her interest in medical education at the National University of Malaysia. She is grateful to Drs. Balasubramaniam, Matthew Gwee and Koh Dow Rhoon, fellow enthusiasts at the National University of Singapore who encouraged and supported her ventures into this field. She also dedicates this book to her late father, Khoo Teng Chye, lifelong educationist and her first teacher. Finally, without the love and support of her children, Ming and En, her contribution to this book would not have been possible.

December 2002
Singapore

Preface

Most ideas about teaching are not new, but not everyone knows the old ideas.

Euclid. Circa 300 BC

Medical education, the science behind the teaching and learning in medicine, has been firmly established as a separate discipline. Parallel to the advancement in medical science, medical education as a discipline has seen tremendous progress. We have reached a phase where we are not limited to understanding what is at fault in our education but we also know *how to correct these faults.* We have progressed from the role of problem-identifier to that of solution-provider.

The beneficial effects of such development are readily evident. Teaching and learning have become more scientific and rigorous, curricula are based on good pedagogical principles, and problem-based and other forms of active and self-directed learning are no longer viewed as an anomaly but are now considered to be the mainstream. There is a strong emphasis on evidence-based education. This is a time of great excitement and opportunity for anyone who is interested in teaching and learning in medicine.

Parallel to its spectacular growth, medical education, as a discipline, has become more specialized. The specialization has taken shape in many forms. There are educators with exclusive interest and expertise in medical education. The discipline itself has become further sub-specialized; there are experts in learning theories, curriculum planning, assessment and evaluation, and clinical education—just to name a few. In most of the leading medical schools, there are autonomous medical education units that lead the educational initiatives. There are several scholarly journals dedicated to medical education which are published regularly and enjoy a good readership base. Moreover, most of the clinical professional journals publish articles on medical education. There are also many authoritative books on various aspects of medical education written by renowned scholars and leaders.

Paradoxically, the rapid development and specialization in medical education has come with a price. The more developed the discipline has become; the more specialized and fragmented have become the books and publications on medical education. Many books are too intimidating and esoteric to meet the needs of general medical teachers. In contrast to the prolific publication trend in specialized aspects of medical education, there is a marked paucity of books written for the general reader in medical education. More importantly, there are few books that are easy to understand, portable, as well as affordable for the individual reader.

The issue of non-availability is evident from our interactions with our colleagues. Frequently, we engage our friends and colleagues in a passionate discussion about medical education and the benefits that they may get from knowing the science of teaching and learning. When we have managed to instill enough interest, our colleagues' response is typical—"It seems medical education is interesting. Can you name a book where I can read more about it?" Our defeat comes now. It is hard to recommend a book about medical education that meets all three criteria of understandability, portability, and affordability.

Therefore, in this simple non-intimidating book, we promise to tell the general medical teachers what they need to know about medical education.

We strive towards making the book a readable, jargon-free, precise yet complete guide to teaching and learning in medicine.

Medical Education as a Discipline

Although medical education benefits from the theory and practice in the field of general education, the unique content, curricular philosophy, teaching and learning methods, and regulatory and social obligation of medicine demand that general education philosophies and practices are applied with careful consideration of these factors. Additional teaching and learning theories and methods are also needed.

The broad discipline of medical education encompasses several sub-divisions including teaching and learning theories, instructional methodology, assessment and evaluation, clinical teaching, and continuing medical education. Besides these, medical education also covers biomedical ethics, health care economics, medical history, and other related fields.

Medical educators are usually medical scientists and clinicians with special interest and expertise in medical education. A medical educator may be someone who is (a) especially skilled in teaching, (b) a person trained in the educational theory and practice in the context of medicine, or (c) an administrator in education. The bulk of medical educators are teaching faculty who have developed supplemental training in the field. The discipline is further enriched by teaching faculty with primary training in education and who have then developed interest in application of educational principles and practice to medical education.

Reasons for Interest in Medical Education

Along with patient care and research, medical teachers are also entrusted by society and medical schools to groom their students to become successful physicians. Almost all medical teachers are given this very significant responsibility without any proper training to become good teachers. Content expertise is a requisite but is not sufficient enough to become good teachers.

Teaching is also a *learnable skill*; this is not an inherent quality that we are born with. Most of us learn the craft of teaching by an arduous, painfully slow and inefficient process of observation of our peers or learning from our own mistakes. Thankfully, the process can be easily improved with proper understanding of a few educational principles and practice of the skills.

We also believe that teaching is a *pleasurable and self-fulfilling* activity. The joy of teaching increases as we master the skills.

Readership of the Book

The profile of the reader that we envision for the book is someone who is interested to know more about medical education but lacks a formal background in pedagogy. This is intended to be a core reading in medical education; not an exhaustive and authoritative reference to the topic.

The primary audience of the book is the general medical teachers from all disciplines and specialties. Both basic science and clinical teachers will benefit from the book. Junior and mid-level teaching staffs will find the book useful as well. It can be used as a faculty resource book for medical teachers. Organizers of medical education workshops may also use this book as a required text.

The book will be useful for teachers and educators from other clinical and para-clinical disciplines including nursing, pharmacy, occupational therapy, and physiotherapy. Although the book is written for medical specialties, educators from other tertiary education will find some of the content relevant and useful to their practice.

Benefits of Reading the Book

The book helps to develop a clear and basic understanding of principles of teaching and learning in medicine. The readers will develop the requisite expertise and skill that are expected of a basic or clinical science teacher including instructional module design, teaching methods, student assessment, and clinical teaching. The readers will also appreciate the changes that are taking place in the field of medical education and the reasons behind the changes.

Most importantly, the book will help the reader to become an effective medical teacher.

Our Approaches

Two discernible approaches are generally noticeable on books on education. The first approach is to focus on the 'why' aspects— a theory based exercise that promotes deep understanding of the topic. The second approach is to target 'how' aspects— demonstrating the practicality and illustrating how the theory is translated into practice. We believe both approaches are valid and have merits on their own and we have tried to strike a balance between the two. Thus, the book not only shows what is important to do but also tells the readers why it is so.

To improve the readability, we have at times simplified the concepts and trimmed what we have thought to be redundant. We recognize this to be a deficiency but a necessary step to keep the content focused on the book's original purposes.

Organization of the Book

The book is divided into several inter-related sections. The preliminary sections provide broad perspectives on medical education including an overview of medical education, historical perspectives, current trends and controversies, and teaching and learning theories. The section on curriculum examines the topic from the perspectives of individual teachers and provides a succinct discussion.

Subsequent sections are organized according to the 'Learning Cycle'—an elementary concept in educational planning. The 'cycle' essentially demonstrates the relationship between the three key elements of teaching and learning: learning objectives, teaching strategies to achieve the objectives, and assessment and evaluation to determine whether the objectives have been fulfilled. The following sections elaborate on each of these elements and cover educational objectives, instructional methodologies including clinical teaching and problem-based learning, and assessment and evaluation. Later sections elaborate on internet and research in medical education.

Each chapter generally starts with a set of objectives. The content evolves around the objectives. Tables and text boxes summarize and reiterate important points. Each chapter ends with a set of key points—a constellation of take-home messages.

The reference section at the end of the each chapter is intentionally kept brief. All the articles and books are easily available—either on the internet or through the local library. Admittedly, there are many more scholarly articles that we mentioned, but those that are not easily available we have not included. The reference section contains two types of articles. The first category includes articles that we have referenced and the second category is 'further reading'—articles that we consider important but not referenced.

In each of the chapter, we have used examples liberally to help readers understand how the concepts may appear in real life. Most of these examples were taken from our own teaching and clinical encounters. But the basic message remains clear enough. There are unavoidable but necessary repetitions in some of the chapters. This is somewhat intentional so that a reader who wants to read a particular chapter is able to do so without much difficulty. Readers are also encouraged to refer frequently to 'Glossary' at the end of the book.

Conventions

Several conventions merit further elaboration. The terms 'we', 'you', 'our', are used to denote medical teachers. We have used the terms teacher, facilitator, faculty, instructor, and so on interchangeably. Students and learners are used interchangeably as well.

To keep a gender-neutral tone and to avoid awkward use of s/he we have used both male and female genders equally. Occasionally, we have also resorted to plural whenever we deemed it appropriate.

The term assessment is used primarily in the context of student assessment and evaluation is used for program evaluation.

We have developed a significant portion of the content from general education resources especially sections on teaching and learning philosophies and teaching strategies. There are convincing reasons for this. General educational resources are much more endowed with rich literature on teaching and learning philosophies and their applications. Although many of these are yet to be tested in medical education, this does not mean these are ineffective or inappropriate; but reflects the relatively new development of medical education as a discipline. Among the general education resources the most helpful was ERIC (Educational Resource Information Clearinghouse, *www.eric.edu*). Readers are urged to use the resource as well.

We know that there are shortcomings and mistakes in the book that we have not realized yet. If you happen to spot one, please drop us an email. We will acknowledge your effort in the next edition.

We are still learning to present the core themes of medical education to readers in a better way. We promise to take seriously any suggestion that readers may have. Meanwhile, we take unconditional responsibility for the remaining lack of clarity and mistakes.

Completion of the book marks the beginning, not the end, of your effort to know the subject. We are confident that you will continue to learn further about medical education, and join us for the betterment of teaching and leaning in medical schools.

Zubair *Amin; zubairamin@hotmail.com*
Khoo Hoon Eng; *bchkhe@nus.edu.sg*
December 2002
Singapore

Contents

Foreword   v

Acknowledgements   vii

Preface   ix

    Medical Education as a Discipline   xi
    Reasons for Interest in Medical Education   xi
    Readership of the Book   xii
    Benefits of Reading the Book   xii
    Our Approaches   xiii
    Organization of the Book   xiii
    Conventions   xiv

Section 1 / Chapter 1   Basic Competencies in
       Medical Teaching   3

    Educational Principles   4
    Curriculum Planning and Design   5
    Instructional Methodologies   6

Student Assessment   7

Conclusion   9

References and Further Readings   10

**Section 2 / Chapter 2   Historical Perspectives in
            Medical Education**   **13**

Asian Medical Schools   15

Deficiencies of the System   16

Call for Reforms   18

What Is Being Done?   20

Role of Medical Education Units   21

Conclusion   22

References and Further Readings   23

Section 3   Educational Concepts and Philosophies

Chapter 3   Teaching and Learning Concepts   **27**

Learner-Centered Learning   28

Surface versus Deep Learning   32

Experiential Learning   34

The Common Themes   37

References and Further Readings   38

Chapter 4   Understanding the Learner   **41**

Conceptual Underpinning   42

Implication of Learning Principles   43

References and Further Readings   46

Chapter 5   Building the Skills of Learning   **49**

Concepts of Metacognition   50

Importance of Metacognition   50

Helping Students Develop Metacognitive Skills . .   50

References and Further Readings   53

Section 4   Curriculum and Learning Cycle

Chapter 6   Curriculum Design and Implementation — 57

Definition . . . . — 58
Strategies for Implementation of Curriculum
Innovations . . . . — 63
References and Further Readings . . . . — 67

Chapter 7   Learning Cycle — 69

Reference and Further Reading . . . . — 71

Section 5   Educational Objectives

Chapter 8   Classification of Educational Objectives — 75

Cognitive Domain . . . . — 78
Psychomotor Domain . . . . — 81
Affective Domain . . . . — 82
References and Further Readings . . . . — 86

Chapter 9   Writing Educational Objectives — 89

The Purpose of Educational Objectives . . . . — 90
Characteristics of Good Educational Objectives . . . — 91
Components of Educational Objectives . . . . — 93
Pitfalls to Avoid . . . . — 94
References and Further Readings . . . . — 95

Section 6   Instructional Methodologies: General

Chapter 10   Overview of Teaching and
Learning Methods — 99

Range of Teaching and Learning Methods . . . . . . — 99
Educational Effectiveness of Teaching and
Learning Methods . . . . — 100

Organization of Chapters   103
References and Further Readings   103

Chapter 11   Making Lecture Effective   105

Advantages   106
Limitations and Concerns   107
Components   108
Ways to Make Lecture More Learner-Centered . . .   110
References and Further Readings   112

Chapter 12   Understanding Small Group   115

Definition   115
Advantages   116
Challenges for Small Group   118
Life Cycle of a Group   119
Types of Group   120
Role and Responsibilities of Tutors in Small Groups   121
References and Further Readings   122

Chapter 13   Case-Based Teaching   123

Definition   123
Educational Rationale   124
Concerns for Case-Based Teaching   125
Variations of Cases for Teaching   126
Case-Selection   126
Preparing the Case for Teaching   127
References and Further Readings   130

Chapter 14   Role-Play   131

Advantages   132
Applications   133
Implementation Considerations   134
The Process   134
Example of Scripts for Role-play:
Counseling Focused   136

Example of Scripts for Role-play:
Clinical Skill Practice 137
References and Further Readings 139

Chapter 15   Questions and Questioning Technique   141

Types of Question 143
Dealing with Students' Wrong Responses 145
Use of Silence 147
References and Further Readings 150

Chapter 16   Providing Effective Feedback   153

Educational Rationale 154
Distinguishing Feedback from Praise and Criticism   154
Nature of Good Feedback 155
Feedback in Group Settings 158
References and Further Readings 159

Section 7   Instructional Methodology: Clinical Teaching

Chapter 17   Conceptual Framework for Clinical Teaching   163

Educational Characteristics of Clinical Teaching . . 163
Precepting in the Context of Clinical Teaching . . . 165
Determining the Learners' Needs 166
Knowledge Base for Clinical Teaching 167
References and Further Readings 170

Chapter 18   Delivery of Clinical Teaching   171

Models of Delivery of Clinical Teaching 172
Teaching Clinical Reasoning Process 175
Common Mistakes During Clinical Teaching 178
References and Further Readings 180

Chapter 19 Assessment of Clinical Competence   **181**

  Concepts of Clinical Competency   181
  Assessing Clinical Competence   182
  Criterion-Based Assessment   185
  References and Further Readings   186

Chapter 20 Teaching Procedural Skills   **189**

  Educational Principles   190
  Broad Categories of Procedural Skills   191
  Less Desirable Way of Teaching Procedural Skill . .   192
  Structured Approach to Procedural Skill Teaching .   192
  Barriers to Learning and Teaching Procedural Skills   196
  References and Further Readings   198

Chapter 21 Teaching Communication Skills   **201**

  The Magnitude of Poor Communication in Medicine   201
  Effects of Good Communication   202
  Teaching Communication in Conventional Ways . .   203
  Communication is a Learnable Skill   204
  Educational Strategies for Teaching
  Communication Skills   204
  References and Further Readings   208

**Section 8 Instructional Methodology:
Problem-Based Learning**

**Chapter 22 Problem-Based Learning (PBL):
Concepts and Rationale**   **213**

  Definition   213
  Historical Overview   215
  Educational Rationale of PBL   215
  Objectives and Outcomes of PBL   216
  Conclusion   217
  References and Further Readings   217

Chapter 23   The PBL Process — 219

Meeting with Case Writers 220
Setting the Pace and Tone of the New Group 220
Session One 221
Session Two 223
References and Further Readings 224

Chapter 24   The Tutor and the Case-Writer — 225

The Tutor's Roles and Responsibilities 226
Practical Skills 227
The PBL Case-Writer 229
References and Further Readings 233

Chapter 25   Student Assessment in PBL — 235

Goals of Student Assessment in PBL 236
Assessment During Tutorial 236
Objective Examinations 237
Assessing Process of PBL—Triple Jump 237
References and Further Readings 238

Chapter 26   Implementation Options of PBL — 241

PBL in New Medical Schools 241
PBL in Existing Medical Schools 242
PBL in Asian Medical Schools: Issues, Challenges,
and Options 245
More Research 246
References and Further Readings 247

Section 9   Assessment and Evaluation

Chapter 27   Overview of Assessment and Evaluation — 251

Concepts of Assessment and Evaluation 252
Value of Needs Assessment 254
Assessor and Assessment Audience 255

The Broad Purposes of Student Assessment   257
Directions in Student Assessment   258
References and Further Readings   260

Chapter 28   Formative and Summative Assessment   261

Formative Assessment   261
Summative Assessment   262
References and Further Readings   265

Chapter 29   Characteristics of Assessment Instruments   267

Validity   267
Reliability   269
Objectivity   270
Practicability   270
Value   271
Errors in Test Items   272
References and Further Readings   274

Chapter 30   Road Map to Student Assessment   275

Factor One: Educational Objectives or Domains . .   276
Factor Two: Level of Knowledge   277
Factor Three: Formative or Summative Assessment   278
Factor Four: Validity of the Instrument   278
Factor Five: Reliability of the Instrument   279
Factor Six: Single Instrument versus
Multiple Instruments   279
References and Further Readings   282

Chapter 31   Multiple Choice Questions   283

Advantages   284
Limitations   285
Components of MCQ   286
Examples of MCQ With Hierarchical
Cognitive Objectives   287
Further Improvements in MCQ   293

Evaluating MCQ 294
References and Further Readings 297

Chapter 32   Essay Questions and Variations   **299**

Advantages 300
Challenges and Limitations 301
Basic Categories of Essay Questions 302
Short Answer Questions (SAQ) 303
Modified Essay Questions (MEQ) 304
References and Further Readings 306

Chapter 33   Oral Examinations   **309**

Advantages 310
Limitations 311
Improving the Validity and Reliability of
Oral Examinations 312
References and Further Readings 315

Chapter 34   Standardized Patient   **317**

Why Do We Need Standardized Patients? 319
Uses 319
Advantages 320
Implementation Considerations 322
References and Further Readings 323

Chapter 35   Portfolio   **325**

What is a Portfolio? 325
The Value of Portfolio 327
Nature of Artifacts in Portfolio 329
Organization of the Portfolio 331
References and Further Readings 333

Chapter 36   Teaching Program Evaluation   **335**

Level One: Reaction 337
Level Two: Learning 338

Level Three: Transfer 339
Level Four: Results 339
References and Further Readings 341

Section 10 / Chapter 37   Internet and Medical Education   345

What is E-Learning? 346
E-learning in Learner-Centered Learning Models . . 346
Design Considerations in E-Learning 350
Learning Objects in E-Learning Models 351
References and Further Readings 354

Section 11 / Chapter 38   Research in Medical Education   357

Nature of Research in Medical Education 358
Difficulties with Interventional Research 361
Value of Qualitative Studies 362
Secondary Researches in Medical Education 363
Framework for Research 364
Priority Research Areas in Medical Education 365
Collaboration in Medical Education Research 366
References and Further Readings 367

Appendix A: Calgary-Cambridge Observation Guide   369

Appendix B: Example of Standardized Patient
Case Script   375

Appendix C: Further Resources   381

Appendix D: Glossary of Terms   385

Index   397

Section 1

Basic Competencies in Medical Teaching

1 Basic Competencies in Medical Teaching

The Latin verb *'docere'* for teach is also the root for the noun 'doctor'. So it would seem that teaching is part of being a doctor. In reality, of course, there are at least three roles for staff in academic medicine: clinical care, research and teaching. All clinical staffs receive training for clinical care in medical school and beyond. Sound training in research can also be provided but is outside the purview of this book. Good teaching also involves skills that must be learnt.

What are these skills? Are there any minimum knowledge base or skills that medical teachers should possess before they become teachers? It is now almost universally agreed that medical teachers should be trained formally in basic educational methods. What has not been firmly established yet are the basic minimum competencies that they should possess. Professional medical or medical education organizations have yet to come up with any firm recommendation in this respect. For example, a question was posed to about 1,000 medical educators belonging to DR-ED listserv newsgroup "What should be the minimum pedagogical competency of medical teachers?" (DR-ED is a forum for discussion and information resource for medical educators. It is maintained by the Office of Medical Education Research and Development (OMERAD) at

Michigan State University, College of Human Medicine.) The question although generated vigorous discussion failed to identify any guideline from professional bodies in this regard (Amin, 02).

Encouragingly, opinions are gradually forming and we have a fair idea about the pedagogical competency of the medical teachers. Moreover, we can extrapolate from other professional higher educational organizations to get a reasonable idea of what medical teachers' pedagogical competency should be.

Therefore, we envision several domains of pedagogical competency and knowledge for basic functioning as medical teachers; (a) a firm understanding of fundamental educational principles as applied to medical education, (b) an understanding of the basics of curriculum, (c) a competency in a range of instructional methodology, and (d) an ability to choose and administer proper assessment methods. We propose that these competencies should be further fine-tuned and be accepted as *essential and universal requisites* for medical teachers. In the following discussion, we elaborate on each of these broad domains and very briefly highlight the key innovations and essential concepts.

Educational Principles

Educational practice should be grounded on sound educational principles. Educational practices that are without sound theoretical construct are unlikely to be effective. While we acknowledge that teaching and learning theories can be dry and boring topics, nevertheless medical teachers need to be conversant with them to understand the rationale for innovations and current trends in medical education. They also need to be fluent in the common terminology that surface frequently in medical education literature.

In a general sense, medical education has been transformed by several powerful theories of learning including learner-centered learning, experiential learning, self-directed learning and deep learning. Congruent with the understanding of learning theories is the better insight of the learning processes of our students or learners. The characterization of our students as learners leads to the concepts of 'adult learner' or the field of andragogy. Finally, another essential concept with practical implications is the skills of learning or metacognition. These three broad fields—learning concepts, adult learning, and skills of learning—provide us the necessary foundation upon which much of the educational activities are undertaken.

Curriculum Planning and Design

The majority of medical teachers spend most of their teaching time directly engaged with the learners. Nevertheless, frequently they are asked to contribute to curriculum planning and evaluation. Thus, the medical teachers should possess a fundamental understanding of curriculum planning and evaluation including how to set educational objectives and prepare and execute an educational plan.

There are several curricular innovations that are of interest to medical teachers. One of the criticisms of the traditional curriculum is the excessive amount of information that medical students are asked to "learn" due to the explosion in knowledge in biomedical sciences. The burden is compounded by repetitions of content over the years. Besides, a great deal of learned content remain unutilized as the students fail to determine the connection between the content and their practical applicability in dealing with patients.

The newer curricula integrate the various disciplines with well-defined objectives. The integration takes shape in various forms: between basic science subjects, between clinical subjects, and between basic and clinical subjects. An immediate effect of such integration is the abandonment of separation between basic and clinical science years. Besides, courses are designed around body systems and functions. Thus, medical teachers' responsibilities include not just imparting facts but also *integrating them and making them relevant to clinical practice*. In addition, they are required to convey necessary professional skills to students.

Instructional Methodologies

The medical teachers' competency in the area of instructional methodology includes effective communication of the course objectives to the students, knowledge and skills about diverse instructional methods, and the ability to choose correct methods of instruction to help students achieve the course objectives. Evidence for effectiveness about specific instructional method comes from myriad sources and includes empirical research and personal and self-reflective research (STLHE, 02).

Thus, it is the sacred responsibility of the medical teacher to maintain the pedagogical competency by taking *active* steps to stay current regarding teaching strategies. Just as he engages in continuing medical education to remain competent professionally, he should engage regularly in reading medical education literature, attend workshops and conferences, experiment with a range of teaching methods, and generally be able to vary his instructional strategies to meet the demand of a specific situation or a particular group of learners.

The response of medical education to the above demands in instructional methodology has resulted in several beneficial changes. First, there are innovations and change in practice to improve already existing 'traditional' and well-established instructional methods such as lectures and other forms of expository learning. The major shift is to make these forms of teaching more active and learner-centered. Secondly, there is expansion of the repository of teaching and learning methods that are available to medical teachers. Medical teachers do not need to confine themselves to a limited number of teaching and learning tools. Small group discussion, brain-storming, role-play, and many others are now regarded as valid instructional methods. They bring variety and can be custom made to suit particular teaching needs.

Thirdly, along with the establishment of new curricula and teaching/training settings, problem-based learning (PBL) and variants have emerged as a convenient and efficient way of delivering learner-centered learning. PBL emphasizes small group and self-directed learning on the part of the student. The content is also more integrated and in some schools where other health care professionals are being taught, training can also be multi-professional.

Thus, the medical teachers' competency in this regards include understanding the core principles and educational rationale of PBL, effective group facilitation skill, student assessment in PBL, and be conversant with various options of PBL implementation.

The fourth area of innovation in instructional methodology is clinical teaching. Unlike the other forms of teaching and learning activities in medicine that share a great deal of similarity with those of general education, clinical teaching is unique to medical education. It involves a number of variables that are peculiar to it including clinical reasoning, patient-based teaching, and a tripartite interaction between students, teachers, and patients.

At the beginning of the early seventies, the predominant hypothesis in understanding the reasoning process was that such reasoning is the result of possession of general 'clinical problem solving skills.' This hypothesis was proven to be wrong and it is believed that generic clinical reasoning process is non-existent (Norman, 2002). What is true is that clinical reasoning is greatly influenced by knowledge that is derived from both formal education as well as from clinical experience. A corollary to this proposition is that with greater understanding of the clinical reasoning process the medical teachers would be able to promote clinical reasoning more effectively.

The other area of improvement in clinical teaching comes in the form of delivering teaching in a time-efficient manner, more effective needs assessment of the learners, and teaching communication and procedural skills to the students. Several innovative models, such as 'microskills', have gained rapid popularity particularly among office-based clinical teachers as an effective way of conducting clinical teaching.

Student Assessment

Assessment is an immensely important activity that all medical teachers are intimately involved with. The stakes in student assessment are high—they are directly related to quality assurance and accreditation of the program. Therefore, it is the duty of the teachers to ensure students assessment to be valid, fair, and linked with the course objectives.

The medical teachers' competency in students assessment includes understanding the basic principles of assessment, recognizing the advantages and disadvantages of various assessment methods, and the ability to choose and implement an assessment instrument that reliably assesses what it intends to assess.

Major innovations that have reshaped student assessments are: (a) more rigorous linking of assessment with program objectives, (b) improvement in validity and reliability of assessment instruments, (c) emphasis on self-assessment and formative assessment, (d) assessment of attitudes and skills along with knowledge, and (e) an attempt to sample actual application of the skills to practice.

Parallel to these developments is a greater appreciation of the *limitations* of student assessment. It is now recognized that tests are snapshots of students' performance in a given time. It may or may not detect the broader aspects of students' competency. To put it more figuratively, it is like punch biopsies of a tumor—we are lucky if we get to make a clear diagnosis with only one biopsy. Nevertheless, the chance of success improves with multiple biopsies and incorporation of *varied* techniques. A realization that leads to the abandonment of one-time testing and development of multiple assessment instruments each with specific strengths.

The range of student assessment instrument now regularly includes multiple choice question, modified and short essay question, oral examination, objective structured clinical assessment, and standardized patients. The student portfolio is being pioneered as an authentic way of documenting students' attitudes and personal attributes (Mathers *et al*, 1999) that are translated into practice. When these are combined judiciously they are much more likely to provide a comprehensive and accurate diagnosis of students' competence.

Conclusion

The introduction of new curricular structures and new methods of teaching, communicating information and student assessment has not been without resistance. Many critics feel that the 'old' methods have worked for so many years, so why should there be any change. Others feel that student-centered methods of teaching where the responsibility is on the student to learn are not viable because the students are not well-prepared. These critics forget that when a teacher teaches, there is no guarantee that the student learns. Thus, the goal of all medical teachers should not be excellence in teaching but rather excellence in ensuring that their students are good at learning. A basic competency in medical pedagogy ensures that this goal is met and learning is meaningful, enjoyable, and usable.

In summary, we have learned that

- Content competency is not enough to become an effective teacher
- The basic minimum competency of medical teacher includes

  - Understanding and determination of application of learning concepts and philosophies
  - Understanding the basics of curriculum planning and implementation
  - Ability to plan and execute an educational program
  - A competency in the range of instructional methodologies
  - An ability to choose and administer proper assessment methods

- The major innovations in medical education include

  - Integrated and flexible curriculum models
  - Problem-based and case-based leaning, greater use of small groups, role-play and other forms of collaborative and group learning
  - Understanding of nature of medical expertise and clinical reasoning

- Development of assessment methods that are more valid and reliable for the intended purpose

References and Further Readings

1. Amin Z. Email to DR-ED list Listserv. 27th June 2002. DR-ED accession number 006839. DR-ED email address: DR-ED@LIST.MSU.EDU.
2. Bland CJ, Schmitz DC, Stritter FT, Henry RC, and Aluise JJ. *Successful Faculty in Academic Medicine: Essential Skills and How to Acquire Them.* 1990. Springer Publication Company, New York, USA.
3. Mathers NJ, Challis MC, Howe AC, and Field NJ. Portfolios in Continuing Medical Education—Effective and Efficient? *Medical Education.* 1999. 33: 521–30.
4. Norman G. Research in Medical Education: Three Decades of Progress. *British Medical Journal.* 2002. 1560–2.
5. Society for Teaching and Learning in Higher Education (STLHE). Ethical Principles in University Teaching. 2002. Canada. Web address: http://www.tss.uoguelph.ca/stlhe/ethics.html. Accessed August 02.
6. Tavanaiepour D, Schwartz PL, and Loten EG. Faculty Opinions about a Revised Pre-Clinical Curriculum. *Medical Education.* 2002. 36: 299–302.

Section 2

Historical Perspectives in Medical Education

2 Historical Perspectives in Medical Education

*Scientists, by reputation, are supposed to be open to ideas, as long as those ideas can be—and are—tested. Let us find faculty who are open to ideas about the management of medical education; let us then test ideas in an atmosphere of mutual trust in our effort to provide the best educational program for the preparation of physicians—which is after all the one mission **unique** to a medical school.*

Abrahamson, 1996

Prior to the 18th century, in Europe and America, the learned study of medicine in the preparation for practice as a physician was limited to members of the social classes that had access to university study. Their patients also tended to be from the same landed and affluent classes. Medicine was studied in university based on the classics of medicine and literature. Latin was predominantly the language of instruction. It was not the same as the practical hands-on work of the surgeons, the pharmacists and other healers.

The situation changed towards the end of the 18th century as advances in science led to the introduction of new subjects such as chemistry, botany and physiology in the university. Even in the traditional medical subjects such as anatomy, materia medica and legal medicine, interest in natural science was increasing. The movement toward practical training in medicine was also gaining momentum and national languages were being used in addition to Latin.

Medical practice itself was also being transformed as medicine, surgery, and therapeutics were drawing together to break down the barriers between physician, surgeons and apothecaries. For example, Loudon wrote that by 1830 the new ideal of a physician in Britain was an all-rounder or a "general practitioner ... who could officiate in all departments of the profession and dispense medicines as well as prescribe."

By the mid-nineteenth century, the programs of study in medical schools still varied from school to school and from country to country but were beginning to show some similarities in structure. The programs included lectures and perhaps demonstrations in the newer sciences, traditional classes in the institutes of medicine, surgery, medical practice, pharmacy, therapeutics and obstetrics and some provisions for clinical or hospital instruction.

The early medical schools in America followed the European model. For example, the first medical school launched in Philadelphia was modeled on the University of Edinburgh because the teachers were graduates from the medical school in Edinburgh. As more and more medical schools were set up in America, many provided excellent training. However, by the end of the 19th century, many others had been set up for profit and standards of training were questionable. As a result, reorganization of American medical education was initiated in several fronts.

The most significant of these initiatives was by Abraham Flexner who was commissioned by the Carnegie Foundation for the Advancement of Teaching. His epic report, 'Medical Education in the United States and Canada', was published in 1910. Interestingly enough, Flexner was not a medial doctor; he was a previously little known headmaster from a private school of Louisville, Kentucky. In his report, he pointed out many shortcomings of the American medical education system and called for higher standard and quality control. He recommended that the medical schools to become integral division of the universities, faculty to be actively involved in original research, and students to participate in active learning through laboratory study and real clinical experience (Ludmerer, 1999).

This system advocated by Flexner included 1–2 years of preclinical basic sciences and 2–3 years of clinical subjects. This was an improvement over the old *ad hoc* system of rather unstructured apprenticeship. Many of the medical schools of lower quality were closed while a new style curriculum was adopted by most of the existing schools. The proposed model was widely accepted in medical schools in North America and beyond and remained so for most part of the twentieth century.

Asian Medical Schools

Colonial powers brought Western medicine to Asia in the 19th century and many Asian medical schools were established in the late nineteenth or early twentieth century. Most of them borrowed and adopted the Western model uncritically. In general, each country had adopted the model from its colonial master. Thus India, Pakistan, Bangladesh, Malaysia, Singapore, and Australia followed the British system. Indochina adopted the French system of admitting students after 12–13 years of primary and secondary school education. The medical curriculum was for 5–6 years with 2–3 years of basic science training and 3–4 years of clinical training. The Indonesian medical schools were largely established after Dutch models with Dutch being the language of instruction. The medical schools in Thailand followed a mixture of both the American and British systems while the Filipinos adopted the American model. The Japanese adopted the German system in the 1860s but after World War Two, came under American influence and adopted its medical education system by introducing a one-year rotating internship and a national licensing examination.

The first school of Western medicine in China was the International Medical School in Guangzhou in 1866. By 1949, there were 56 medical colleges and faculties in China. Medical education was disrupted during the Cultural Revolution and colleges only reopened in 1975. By 1982, there were 116 medical colleges with approximately 30,000 new students each year enrolled in Western medicine, traditional Chinese medicine and other health science programs.

In Asia, most of the medical schools were established and maintained by the government. Although the government control has hindered change and adaptation of newer innovations in the medical schools, arguably the control also has the salutary effect of maintaining a certain degree of standards. In recent years, the central control has been gradually weakening in part due to establishment of many private medical schools. Many of these medical schools are proprietary and profit-driven without any meaningful link to reputed universities. Ironically this trend of establishing decentralized and often profit-driven medical school is remarkably similar to situations that prompted medical education reform by Flexner almost 100 years ago.

The challenges facing medical education in Asia are similar across different countries. The learning process is still problematic with large classes and limited opportunities for students to pursue independent learning or electives. Assessment system is antiquated and deficient in requisite validity and reliability. Medical schools in many countries are still struggling to revitalize their medical education system and realign it with the needs and priorities of the society. Encouragingly there is a positive trend towards systematic approach to medical education with openness and eagerness that was never seen before.

Deficiencies of the System

By the end of the 20th century, the Flexnerian system had been adopted worldwide as one way of balancing a sound scientific basis with clinical education. It established a standard in medical education with focus on quality control and served the medical schools for over a century.

However, in recent years it has been realized that the model needs to be changed to meet the newer and changing roles of medical schools. The criticisms are directed at several fronts. The Flexnerian model has a clear and artificial separation between basic sciences and clinical sciences. As a result, there is a lack of continuity and unnecessary repetitions of the contents. Much of the knowledge learned during the basic science years become lost in clinical years as their practical applications remain unclear to the students.

The medical schools were also part of a university system with strong orientation towards research. Such a system had led to tremendous advances in medical research but not for medical education. Both basic and clinical sciences had become more focused on research while the content of the curriculum had become more specialized. Medical educational programs became more inward-looking towards increasingly narrow disciplines. Overall, the end result was a serious mismatch between the profile of the doctors being trained and the needs of the community.

Basic science versus clinical training

Worldwide, in the medical schools following the Western style curriculum, the balance between acquiring scientific biomedical theories and learning clinical skills has been swinging back and forth. Unfortunately, many medical schools do not appear to have a clear educational mission. They have not clearly stated the answers to several critical questions. What should the primary focus of medical education be? Should it be the needs of the patient or the demands for scientific rigor? Where should learning take place—the library or the lecture hall or the clinic? Do the medical schools want to train clinical practitioners or researchers or both?

The struggle between these conflicting and sometimes irreconcilable demands and the debate about what constitutes quality in medical education has been between two groups. On one side are those who believe that the quality of doctors would be jeopardized by a lack of scientific rigor. Therefore they have advocated the strengthening of basic science in the medical school curriculum by increasing its content. As advances in biomedical knowledge exploded exponentially, one of the consequences was therefore to place emphasis on the teacher as the expert who transmitted information via didactic lectures. Curricula were often poorly coordinated as individual basic science departments sought to teach as much as possible to the medical student without indicating the relevance of the science to clinical practice. By the time the student reached the clinical disciplines, much of the basic science knowledge that had been memorized in the earlier years was forgotten.

On the other side of the debate are those who believe that medical education should serve the needs of the community and the patient. Thus, emphasis should be placed in the training of medical practitioners by increased exposure to clinical training including primary care and communication skills, ethics, preventive medicine and health maintenance. These contradictions serve to emphasize that medical school decision–makers have to be clear about what type of doctors they want to train.

Call for Reforms

As criticisms became more widespread, curricular reforms were instituted worldwide. Several international organizations such as WHO, the World Federation for Medical Education and the Network of Community-Oriented Educational Institutions for Health Sciences (now known as The Network: Towards Unity for Health) publicized the need to reform medical curricula to fit the society in which the medical school is situated.

Recommendations from UK

In 1993, the General Medical Council (GMC) in the UK recommended that the aim of the undergraduate medical course should be to produce doctors with the attitudes toward medicine and learning which would fit them for their future professional careers and self-directed life-long learning. Thus, the medical curriculum should include courses that emphasize compassion, communication skills, and appropriate behavior and allow for independent learning. The GMC identified two major reforms as critical factors to achieve the goals: (a) reduction of factual overload and (b) promotion of self-education, critical thinking and evaluation of scientific evidence. The content of the curriculum should be defined and limited while the teaching/learning processes should be changed to a more active style. Many of the reforms should also target at making the basic sciences more relevant to the practice of medicine.

Recommendations from USA

The Johnson Wood report in 1992 made several important recommendations that have been accepted by many medical schools worldwide too. Some of these recommendations are similar to recommendations from other professional bodies. Firstly, it urged more integration of the basic science throughout the entire curriculum rather than confining it to the first 2–3 years. So there should be more interdisciplinary and interdepartmental courses in which students in their early years encounter clinical problems that require knowledge of basic sciences. This should be carried forward to their clinical training years when they learn to use their basic science knowledge to solve clinical problems.

The second recommendation was to incorporate the behavioral and social aspects of health and disease including statistics, information sciences, and ethics into the curriculum. Familiarity with these topics would prepare the medical graduate to practice health promotion and disease prevention as well as allow the doctor to access new medical knowledge as part of life-long learning.

The third recommendation involved the extension of clinical training beyond the tertiary-care hospitals that had become the main training environment of most medical schools. Thus, students should be exposed to ambulatory care settings, community or rural hospitals, general practitioner clinics, nursing homes and hospices. Such training would allow the students to see patients in different settings and understand the role and need for primary care.

The fourth recommendation covered the area of assessment of medical students. It was suggested that just as the curriculum should be interdisciplinary and inter-departmental, methods of assessment should also be integrated. Both basic science and clinical staffs should therefore be involved in preparing the same examinations. Methods used to assess students' achievements can greatly influence their learning. Thus with the emphasis on active and student-centered learning, evaluation methods should also be congruent with these goals.

In order for curricular reforms to be successful, the last recommendation was to create a central coordinating authority within the medical school for implementing the changes. Thus, this authority would be responsible for planning, implementing, monitoring, evaluating and reviewing the curriculum, revising it as necessary and rewarding teaching excellence.

What Is Being Done?

The best curriculum is the one that produces a graduate who matches the mission statement of the medical school. For the 21st century, who will be a good physician? There is no right answer but most schools agree that he/she should be someone who would promote the health of all people, be aware of equity in health care, deliver health services in humane and cost-effective manner, be able to carry out his learning independently and throughout his professional life, and have high moral and ethical standard that is reflective of societal aspirations. With these realizations many medical schools have re-visited at their existing mission statements and in the absence of such mission statements forced to create one.

To achieve the stated mission statements or goals, most medical schools have also revised their curriculum. One of the most evident and increasingly widespread innovation is the introduction of the problem-based learning method that was first practiced at McMaster University in 1969. The use of standardized patients for clinical teaching and assessment is another interesting development. Thus, the licensing boards in several countries have already introduced the use of standardized patients in their examinations. A third trend is the increasing use of ambulatory-care settings for medical students' clinical learning experiences. Finally, almost all curricula now strive towards integration of basic science with clinical training.

For example, the Faculty of Medicine at National University of Singapore has the following educational objectives for its new curriculum introduced in 1999. The graduate should be able to understand and apply the scientific basis of medicine to the diagnosis, management and prevention of disease and to the maintenance of health, develop skills for continual and self-directed learning, observe the professions' ethical obligations, demonstrate appropriate behavior, and communicate effectively with patients, collaborators and colleagues.

Several fundamental changes in teaching and learning experiences were necessary to achieve the stated objectives. The old curriculum was highly teacher-centered, lecture-based and discipline-oriented. The new curriculum has been changed to become more student-centered, integrated, interactive and faculty-directed. The new five-year curriculum was integrated across the basic science as well as with the clinical disciplines. The content was *reduced* and special study modules were incorporated into the first four years of the curriculum to allow for more independent learning. Students were introduced to some basic elements of patient care in the first year. PBL was used as method for 20% of curriculum time. The time allocated to training in community health clinics was increased. Determination of academic content and student assessment came under the aegis of a central curriculum committee chaired by a Vice-Dean rather than individual departments. A medical education unit was also set up to institute faculty development and conduct research in medical education.

Role of Medical Education Units

Sustaining medical education is not a minor undertaking and it takes professional educational expertise to accomplish the necessary tasks. Most medical schools that are serious about medical education have established a medical education unit or its equivalent. Among 130 schools of medicine in the USA and Canada, 111 schools have a Medical Education Unit (MEU). Sixty-three of these 111 MEU have been established in the last decade (1990–2000) (Anderson, 2000).

The MEU plays a major role in faculty development. It trains staff in medical pedagogy, clinical teaching, student assessment, and program evaluation. The MEU also participates in training medical students in group dynamics, small group learning activities and PBL. MEU helps in the development and monitoring of curriculum by providing appropriate design and innovations and assists curriculum committees in instructional methods, clinical teaching, and student assessment.

Last but not least, MEU plays a vital role in medical education research and the search for evidence for better practices. Thus, the MEU can function as a think-tank to lead research and scholarship in diverse aspects of medical education. Participation in the activities of a medical education unit is a useful way for the keen basic scientists or clinical staffs to contribute positively to medical education in their own medical school.

Conclusion

Medical education will evolve continually to become more relevant for the changing needs of society and to adjust to the explosion of biomedical scientific knowledge. Medical teachers should be more proactive in their own training in educational methods that emphasize active learning and foster self-directed learning in the student.

In summary, we have learned that

- Modern medical curricula design has been a struggle between the theory and the practice of medicine
- The model proposed by Flexner in the 1920s tried to strike a balance with 2 years of pre-clinical basic science training

followed by 2–3 years of clinical training and was adopted by medical schools worldwide

- Flexnerian model has drawn criticisms for artificial separation of basic science and clinical practice
- Recent reforms in medical education includes greater emphasis on active and self-directed learning, across the board integration of disciplines, and generally a more humanistic and need-based approach to medical education
- Many such reform processes require professional expertise from medical educators and strong commitment from the medical schools for teaching faculty development

References and Further Readings

1. Abrahamson S. *Essays on Medical Education*. University Press of America, Inc. 1996 Maryland. p 113. USA.
2. Anderson B. A Snapshot of Medical Students' Education at The Beginning of The 21st Century: Report from 130 Schools. *Academic Medicine*. 2000. 75: 9. Supplement (September).
3. Bonner TN. *Becoming a Physician*. Johns Hopkins University Press. 1995 Paperback edition. 2000. Baltimore. Maryland, USA.
4. Bowers JZ, Hess JW, and Sivin N. (Editors). *Science and Medicine in Twentieth-Century China*. Research and Education: Center for Chinese Studies. 1988. Ann Arbor. University of Michigan. USA.
5. Choa GH (editor). Recent Developments in Medical Education; Proceedings of the Seminar on Recent Developments in Medical Education held at The Chinese University of Hong Kong on July 6–7, 1978. 1979. The Chinese University Press. Hong Kong.
6. Flexner A. *Medical Education in the United States and Canada*. Carnegie Foundation for the Advancement of Teaching. 1910. Bulletin Number 4. New York, USA.
7. Lim KA (editor). Medical Education in Southeast Asia: A Seminar Report. ASAIHL Seminar on Medical Education in Southeast Asian Universities (University of Singapore: 1970);

Association of Southeast Asian Institutions of Higher Learning, Bangkok, Thailand.

8. Loudon I. *Medical Care and the General Practitioner:1750–1850.* 1986. Clarendon Press, Oxford. pp 194–195.

9. Ludmerer K. *Time to Heal: American Medical Education from the Turn of the Century to the Managed Care Era.* 1999. Oxford University Press. New York, NY, USA.

10. Marston RQ and Jones RM. (editors) Medical Education in Transition Commission on Medical Education. 1992. The Sciences of Medical Practice: Robert Wood Johnson Foundation, Princeton, N.J., USA.

11. Towle A. The Aims of the Curriculum: Education for Health Needs in 2000 and Beyond. In: Jolly B. and Rees L. (editors). 1998. *Medical Education in the Millennium.* Oxford University Press.

Educational Concepts and Philosophies

3 Teaching and Learning Concepts

With this chapter, we advance towards building-up a basic understanding of the relevance of teaching and learning concepts and principles together with their applications in medical education. While there are many such concepts, we confine our discussion to a few selected and important ones. Other concepts are discussed where relevant to enable us to establish a direct connection between the concepts with their practical applications.

In this chapter, our tasks are to

- Discuss and explain fundamental educational principles behind learner-centered learning, deep learning, and experiential model of learning
- Determine and illustrate their applications in the context of medical education
- Identify what is our current educational status and where we ought to be
- Propose changes in the educational environment that are necessary to implement learner-centered learning, deep learning, and experiential learning

There are several compelling reasons to understand these concepts. They are essential elements that explain the educational phenomena in a scientific and logical manner. Most teaching and learning models that we will be discussing in the subsequent chapters are based on these concepts and the terms will surface recurrently. Moreover, an appreciation of these concepts is required to convince us of the need for changes in medical education.

We urge you not to view the concepts as competing theses. They are valid in explaining elements and phenomena in education. Also, there is no 'unified' theory that can singularly explain every aspect of teaching and learning.

Concepts are presented here in a *simplified and abbreviated* manner. At times, there are oversimplifications to keep the reading easy. The concepts are based on the original work of renowned educational psychologists including Kolb, Gibbs and Habeshaw, Ashcroft and Foreman-Peck, and Flavell. Interested readers are urged to consult their definitive works.

Learner-Centered Learning

> *Personally, I'm always ready to learn, although I do not always like being taught.*
>
> Winston Churchill

Learner-centered or student-centered learning is one of the most widely used terms in contemporary medical education. The influence of learner-centered learning is more far-flung than we realize. The learner-centered learning model has reshaped almost all aspects of medical education. Curriculum planning, instructional models, student assessment, application of internet technology, even classroom design are inspired by this concept. The concept is relevant to all players in medical education—students, teachers, administrators, policy makers, and the public.

Why is learner-centered learning so important?

The emergence of learner-centered approaches in medical education is, at least in part, a response to the explosion of knowledge in medicine. The medical curriculum has grown tremendously both in terms of depth and content coverage. Information is fast changing—it is estimated that medical knowledge doubles in every five years. What is being taught in medical school loses its relevance substantially during the practice years. Also, the complexity of medical knowledge necessitates more than just factual knowledge retention. It demands more analytical ability and problem-solving skills throughout the doctor's professional life.

The traditional medical schools' curricula and instructional methods are heavily teacher-dominated and student-passive processes. Students are often indifferent to their learning and unable to carry out their learning independently. Independent learning is a critical attribute needed for enhancing analytical and problem solving abilities as well as to continue learning throughout life. Proponents of learner-centered learning believe that this method of learning delivers what traditional curricula and instructional methods have failed to achieve. The learner-centered model nurtures and prepares the learners to be independent and self-reliant in their learning, efficient and more responsive to the needs of the fast-changing and ever-demanding field of medicine. It also emphasizes the *process of learning* along with the content.

Theoretical foundation

Two dominant theories in education are crucial in our understanding of the learner-centered learning approach. The earlier model of teaching and learning was proposed by Skinner and known as the *instructivist* (from original verb 'instruction') theory. This model emphasizes the *role of instruction* on students' learning—learning is the direct result of instruction. Because instruction is a significant way of teaching and learning, students are *dictated* in their learning endeavor. The learning activities are *provided* with structured lectures, textbooks, and are progressively exposed to graded difficulty of problems. Good results act as a stimulus for further learning. Teachers reinforce learning by way of feedback, review, and repeated practice (Fardouly, 01).

The newer model is known as *constructivist* (from original verb 'construction') theory that forms the basis of the learner-centered approach. Constructivist theory emphasizes the importance of *active and reflective nature of learning and the learner*. This theory places greater importance on the learners' internal mental state. Motivation for learning comes from the learners themselves. Learners decide on their *own* learning goals. Their pursuit for knowledge is supported from interactions with others. Thus, learning is an individual as well as a *social and collaborative process*. The information obtained from the learning process is internalized and learners transform the information in a way that makes new sense to them. The teacher's role is mostly as a facilitator—he provides necessary help and direction to the learners to learn. Strategies for learning include case- and problem-based learning, projects, peer teaching, and group work (Fardouly, 01). Learning activities greatly encourage the learners to develop the *skills for learning*—a term formally known as metacognition (Flavel, 1970).

Learner-centered learning is a *shared and collaborative activity* between the teachers and the students. Teachers help the students to learn. This marks a giant-step forward from the traditional assigned roles of teachers and students where 'teachers teach and students learn.' In learner-centered learning, teaching and learning are a joint exercise that benefits from the combined responsibility.

The opposing paradigm of teacher-dominated versus learner-centered approach is eloquently expressed as 'push versus pull' approaches. In the traditional model, the learning contents are pushed to the learners with little or no options of choice and selection. Whereas in learner-centered learning models, the learners enjoy a fair degree of autonomy that allows them to decide and choose the necessary contents and other learning activities.

Features of Learner-centered Learning

- Learning is active and self-directed
- Active reflection and discovery enhance the learning
- Motivation to learn is intrinsic
- Learning is an individual as well as a social and collaborative activity
- Teachers act as a facilitator
- Learning is a shared and joint activity between the teacher and student
- Learner determines (with support from teachers) own goals, methods of achieving the goals, and assessment process
- Skills of learning improve the learning

Barriers to implementation

As learner-centered learning is a collaborative activity, *both* students and teachers need education and training about the process. Teachers hesitate as they wrongfully perceive the concept as inherently unstructured, disorganized, and a threat to their control over the classroom. Moreover, teachers need to be trained to become effective facilitators—a role that many have not had prior experience with. Students feel vulnerable, as they are not trained in the skills of learning. They need to know how learner-centered learning works, their expanded responsibility and role, and generally how to be an effective learner in this context.

Opponents of the learner-centered learning model also argue that many of the higher order cognitive processes that are championed by this concept are difficult to assess, or not assessed at all, by the conventional assessment techniques. This is a valid concern that can be addressed with incorporation of newer assessment techniques and improvement of existing ones.

What do we need to do to promote learner-centered learning?

Arguably, promotion and implementation of learner-centered learning is an undertaking that is to be carried out at the medical school level. But, while that is waiting to happen what can we do at the *individual tutor level* to promote learner-centered learning? Is it possible or practical?

Reassuringly, the practice of learner-centered learning does not have to be a grand affair. Within the microcosm of the classroom and clinical teaching, we can easily practice simple steps that would go a long way towards the promotion of learner-centered learning.

Promoting Learner-Centered Learning at Individual Level

- Be less directive, be more facilitative
- Emphasize the process of learning along with content
- Encourage peer teaching, small group discussion, case-based teaching
- Make lecture interactive
- Help learners decide on need-driven goals
- Teach principles, not esotericism, with wider appeals and applications
- Promote self-reflection and self-assessment
- Introduce variations to teaching and learning methods

Surface versus Deep Learning

The concept of surface versus deep learning parallels the development of learner-centered learning and is credited to Gibbs (1992). Gibbs emphasizes the importance of outcome of learning in deciding what approach learners may take in their learning endeavor.

Surface learning is a form of *superficial learning* that is confined to knowledge acquisition only. The outcomes of such learning activities are primarily limited to memorization of the facts and reproduction of these facts at the desired time. The process discourages the learner from venturing beyond knowledge acquisition and there is no attempt to obtain deeper understanding or meaning of the facts. The motivation of surface learning is often extrinsic—typically the desire to clear the hurdles of examinations. The performance at such examinations is determined by the ability of the learners to reproduce the memorized materials. As such, surface learning does not promote the desirable attributes of learning processes such as knowledge application, analysis, and critical thinking (Gibbs, 1992; Ashcroft and Foreman-Peck, 1994).

In contrast, deep learning seeks to understand the *deeper meaning of knowledge*. It involves understanding the concepts, principles, and their possible applications. As learners progress through the process of deep learning, they interpret the newly acquired knowledge in the light of their prior experience and knowledge and typically assign new meaning to it. This process of internalization of knowledge imparts permanence to it. The motivation of deep learning is often *internal*—self-satisfaction upon understanding a concept and the joy of discovering the applicability of the knowledge. The process of deep learning helps promote many wholesome attributes such as application, analysis, and critical thinking (Gibbs, 1992; Ashcroft and Foreman-Peck, 1994).

Surface learning and deep learning are not mutually exclusive and it is possible for the two to coexist. Which type of learning the learners will pursue very much depends on the prior educational experiences of the learners and nature of the educational tasks. For example, prior success and satisfaction with deep learning are strong motivating factors for subsequent choice of deep learning. The teachers also play a vital role in the decision process by determining the nature of the tasks and setting up their expectations of the students.

How do we promote deep learning in our students? Gibbs proposes several strategies for promotion of deep learning. Many of these strategies are remarkably similar to suggestions that are made for promotion of other desirable learning atmosphere such as learner-centered learning and experiential learning. In essence, deep learning is more likely to take place in situations where

- The motivation for learning is intrinsic, as opposed to extrinsic such as examinations and tests
- Personal development is valued and expected
- Active learning, such as problem- and project-based learning, is practiced and promoted
- There are ample opportunities for group and collaborative work
- Self-exploration is promoted
- Knowledge is presented in a whole and integrated fashion rather than in fragments

---

Attributes that Promote Deep Learning

- Intrinsic motivation
- Personal and professional development
- Active learning
- Group and collaborative work
- Self-exploration, discovery, and reflection
- Integrated concepts and curriculum
- Match between assessment and learning objectives

Barriers to Deep Learning

- Extrinsic motivation
- Learning and teaching for examination
- Passive learning
- Learning in isolation
- Fragmentation of knowledge

Experiential Learning

Kolb (1984) in his landmark theory highlights the importance of *life experience* in learning. His theory, experiential learning theory (from experience), is important in the understanding of adult learning activities, continuing life-long learning, and many of the informal learning activities in which we are engaged.

The experiential learning theory proposes that learning is the result of four inter-related activities that progress sequentially and constitute a cycle. The central premise of the theory is based on the observation that learning largely results from incorporation of life experiences into one's own thinking. Thus, learning is determined by and benefits from assimilation and integration of life-experiences.

The first stage of Kolb's learning cycle is concrete experience. The learners' responsibility starts with engaging in the life experience. Later, the learners observe and reflect on the experience to understand the meaning of the event. The observation and reflection are essential to convert the experience into meaningful learning activities. With the help of reflection, the learners develop some concepts and general principles. In the final stage, they apply the general concepts and principles into new situations. And, the cycle of experimentation, reflection, development of general principles, and application into new situations continues (Fig. 1).

To illustrate and simplify the concept further, let us imagine ourselves as physicians involved in treating hypertensive patients. At the beginning, we engage ourselves with real experience (Step One: Experience) by providing anti-hypertensive medications to the patients. After treating several patients, we start the process of observation where we collect data about the effects of the treatment. We realize that some of the patients benefited as expected but others did not. We try to understand the reasons for success and failure in the treatment. In other words, we engage ourselves in reflection (Step Two: Observation and reflection). After some brain-storming we may see a pattern and develop some general principles with regards to the treatment. We may be able to identify certain characteristics of the patients that predict the most suitable modality of treatment for them (Step Three: General principles). Once we are equipped with the new knowledge, we apply these

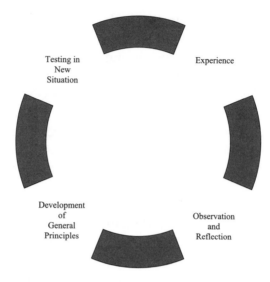

Testing in
New
Situation

Experience

Development
of
General
Principles

Observation
and
Reflection

Fig. 1. The Kolb's experiential learning cycle.

to new patients (Step Four: Testing in new situations). The cycle continues and repeats itself.

How can we apply Kolb's learning model to our teaching and learning? Two immediate and proximate applications of this model are to improve (a) our own teaching and (b) our students' learning. The experiential model is a powerful tool to reflect on and improve our own teaching. Let us illustrate an example how we can apply this model in our own context. Suppose, recently we have learned about interactive lecturing and want to apply some of the recommendations. After several lectures, we realize that not all the tips work in every situation. Sometimes, we are able to engage learners into an energetic discussion, while at other times we just fail to spark a discussion. We may be able to recognize patterns of situations where the recommendations are likely to work and where they generally fail. We may even develop some general principles like 'Questions should be probing and interesting enough for the students' or 'I should discuss what is important for my students to learn, not what is easy to teach'. Equipped with these newly learned general principles, we may restructure our lecture. And the cycle repeats itself.

In a similar manner we can apply the Kolb's learning model among our students to improve their learning. The learning principles behind self-assessment and portfolio-based learning are substantially derived from experiential learning model. We will elaborate on these in subsequent chapters.

The Common Themes

An intelligent reader can clearly detect common threads among the learning concepts and principles. In the following scheme, we have chosen several paired themes; the left-hand side represents less desirable ones, the right-hand side represents where we should be. Look at the scheme carefully and think for a few minutes. For each pair, where do you think your own situation is? Is it more towards the left or towards the right? What kind of changes do you propose at the individual teacher's level that would move the situation more towards the right? What kind of policy changes do you think your medical school should undertake?

Teacher-Centered Teaching	$\longrightarrow$	Learner-Centered Learning
Passive Learning	$\longrightarrow$	Active Learning
Motivation: Examination	$\longrightarrow$	Motivation: Learning
Learning in Isolation	$\longrightarrow$	Group and Collaborative Learning
Fragmentation of Knowledge	$\longrightarrow$	Integration of Knowledge
Predominance of Lecture	$\longrightarrow$	Varied Instructional Methods
Rote Memory	$\longrightarrow$	Comprehension, Application, and Problem Solving
Teacher Directed Assessment	$\longrightarrow$	Incorporation of Self and Peer Assessment

Learner-centered and other forms of learning models that we have discussed are *not* unstructured undertakings. Neither are they a constellation of disjointed and random activities. On the contrary, these models are based on sound educational principles that demand rigor in planning and execution. They bring rational order to the way teaching and learning is pursued.

In summary, the important concepts that we have learned are

- Learner-centered learning is a form of active and reflective learning that is initiated and maintained by the learners' intrinsic motivation to learn
- Group activity and collaboration enhance the learning
- Strategies for learner-centered learning include case-based, project-based, and problem-based learning
- Development of skills for learning is vital for learner-centered learning to be successful
- Surface learning is practiced in situations where motivation for learning is extrinsic. Whereas, in deep learning, the motivation is internal—the desire of the individual to understand and apply what he has learnt
- Experiential learning emphasizes sequential progression of experimentation, observation and reflection, development of general principles, and testing the principles in new situations
- Experiential learning can be applied to improve our own teaching as well as students' learning

References and Further Readings

1. Ashcroft K and Foreman-Peck L. *Managing Teaching and Learning in Further and Higher Education*. 1994. The Falmer Press. London. UK.
2. Fardouly N. *Principle of Instructional Design and Adult Learning: Learner-Centered Teaching Strategy*. Faculty of Built Environment. University of New South Wales. Australia. March, 2001. Web address: http://www.fbe.unsw.edu.au/Learning/ instruction-aldesign/, accessed May 2002.

3. Flavell JH. Metacognition and Cognitive Monitoring: A New Era of Cognitive-Developmental Monitoring. *American Psychologist*. 1979. 34: 906–11.
4. Gibbs G and Habeshaw T. *Preparing to Teach: An Introduction to Effective Teaching in Higher Education*. Technical and Educational Services. Bristol. UK.
5. Kolb DA. *Experiential Learning*. Prantice Hall. Chicago. IL. USA.
6. Stage FK, Muller PA, Kinzie J, and Simmons A. Creating Learning Centered Classrooms. What Does Learning Theory Have To Say? *ERIC Digest*. 1998 ERIC Clearinghouse on Higher Education, Washington, DC ERIC_NO: ED422777.

4 Understanding the Learner

In the earlier chapter, we have learned about the basic concepts and premises in teaching and learning. In this chapter, we focus on the practical implications of those in dealing with 'adult learner.' The term adult learner, in this context, is used to denote the psychological and intellectual maturity rather than chronological age of an individual. Thus, both we, as teachers, and the medical students are adult learners and the principles apply to our own learning situations as well to our students.

In this chapter, our tasks are to

- Discuss the concepts of adult learners
- Recognize their special learning needs and characteristics
- Propose educational features that are more likely to be successful with them

The principles of adult learning evolve around the basic premise that adult learners have special learning characteristics. It is believed that adults are not captive learners; if the contents, instructional methods, and evaluation processes do not conform to their liking and needs they lose enthusiasm for learning (Imel, 1994).

The concepts of adult learning, in large part, are credited to revered educationist Malcolm Knowles who in the early fifties proposed several learning characteristics to describe adult learners. Part of Knowles' theory builds upon the works of famous behavioral psychologists Piaget and Erikson. Knowles suggested a new model of adult learning that distinguishes between teacher-centered and learner-centered teaching and learning models. He fervently advocated the learner-centered model as the preferred learning strategy for adults. His proposed model is known as the andragogical model and study of adult learning is known as andragogy.

Conceptual Underpinning

The andragogical model underwent expansion and advancement around several key concepts. Understandably, fundamental premises and assumption of these concepts are very much akin to other learning models that we have discussed and there is substantial overlap.

- *Self-directed learning*: Self-directed learning proposes that adults prefer to take control of their own learning. The process encompasses every aspect of learning in adults. Adults set their own learning goals, locate appropriate material and human resources, decide on the learning methods to use, and evaluate their own progress. The teacher's role is that of a resource person and facilitator.
- *Critical reflection*: Critical reflection is believed to be uniquely an adult learning phenomenon that is also bolstered by behavioral psychology. Critical reflection is the outcome of an ongoing struggle where the adults deliberately explore a particular event with an attempt to learn and improve upon. In the process adults constantly challenge, revise, and replace older beliefs and develop an alternate viewpoint of life.
- *Learning from experience*: Life experience is crucial to adult learning. Adults drawn into an educational process possess

extensive experience. It is proposed that 'experience is the adult learner's living textbook' and that adult education is, therefore, 'a continuing process of evaluating experiences.' (Lindeman, 1926). An extension of this theme is that adult teaching should be grounded on adults' experiences and these experiences represent valuable educational resources.

- *Learning to learn*: Adults thrive to know how to learn i.e. to become skilled at learning in a range of different situations and through a range of different styles. In broader terms, it means that adults possess a self-conscious awareness of how it is they come to know what they know. They ceaselessly struggle to create an awareness of the reasoning, assumptions, evidence and justifications that underlie their beliefs that something is true (Brookfield, 1995).

Implication of Learning Principles

The implications of adult learning theory in medical education are far-reaching. It applies to medical students, trainee doctors, and physicians in practice. All phases of teaching and learning—content identification, objective determination, instructional model planning, and program evaluation, can be shaped according to this andragogical model. Although each individual adult is unique, certain generalizations are also possible that would help teachers in effective planning of educational activities for adults.

Assessing learners' needs: A good education program starts with defining the tasks that are directly linked with the learners' needs. Needs assessment also helps in determining the quantity and the extent of directions that the adult learners would require during an educational program. Through the needs assessment, adults can identify their problem areas among the course topics to determine the starting point of their learning. Teachers should encourage the adult learners to get involved in their own needs assessment as this is more likely to result in meaningful partnership with the teacher.

Creating an effective adult learning environment: A good adult learning environment addresses both the physical and psychological needs of the learners. While physical needs are easily met, psychological needs commonly assume complex dimensions and are more difficult to address. Adults may feel threatened from the educational process; they are often anxious learners who always remain vigilant for fear of appearing naive or exposing themselves. Neutralizing their fear is one of the key tasks of the teachers. Conversely, they should not feel so safe that they do not question their current assumptions or are not challenged in other ways (Imel, 1994). The trick is to create a balanced environment where adults *feel safe but intellectually challenged*.

Promotion of participatory learning: Benefits of participatory learning include capitalization of experiences and prior learning of participants, breaking the monotony of routine classroom, and cultivation of self-directed learning. Well-designed group work is one of the suggested strategies in participatory learning and achievable in both small group and large group settings. Group activities are possible in a short-term process such as brainstorming and can be formed for ongoing longer projects as well.

Promotion of individual learning: Adults prefer problem or task oriented approach to learning over subject oriented approach. This stems from the fact that adults come to an educational program with pre-defined needs of their own that they can relate to in their real life. Whenever possible, teacher should support and nurture opportunities for individual problem solving. They should assist and assign them with their own tasks and help them towards achieving that.

Motivation: Adults attend an educational program either from internal motivation (e.g. needs to learn a new procedural skill) or from influence of external factors (e.g. a rise in salary or prospect of promotion). Internal motivations are much stronger and sustainable. The best way to motivate adult learners is simply to *enhance their reasons* (e.g. self-realization that a new skill is required) and *to remove the barriers*. Instructors should also be aware of the motivating factors and be prepared to cultivate those during the program.

Assessment: Although many adult learning activities may not need formal assessment, it is useful to provide adult learners ways to identify and assess their own resources, abilities and knowledge. When formal assessment is required suggested strategies include de-emphasizing the traditional authority role and emphasizing the learner's role as an autonomous, responsible adult (Kopp).

According to Rogers, 'Learning is part of a circuit that is one of life's fundamental pleasures: the [teachers'] role is to keep the current flowing.' (Roger, 1989). Teachers are more likely to succeed with adult learners if they take into account adult learning characteristics and apply those principles into practice. The key is to engage the adults as partners by providing direction and support during their learning.

In summary, the important concepts that we learned are

- Adults prefer learner-centered learning model as this provides greater autonomy and control over their learning
- Adults learning is supported by proper utilization of reflective process and development of learning skills
- Life experience is an important determinant of adult learning
- Adults need to feel safe but challenged in a learning situation
- Participatory and group learning are immensely beneficial for adult learners

Characteristics of Adult Learners

- Adults learn what they consider is important
- Adults tend to be self-directing
- Adults have a rich reservoir of experience that serves as a resource for learning
- Adults prefer task- or problem-centered orientation to learning as opposed to a subject-matter orientation
- Adults are generally motivated to learn due to intrinsic factors
- Adults like to be treated as adults and will demand so
- Adults generally want immediate applications of new information or skills to current problems or situations
- Adults want to determine not only what they learn but also to identify and establish their own assessment techniques

(Developed in part and with modification from Susan Imel. Guidelines for Working with Adult Learners. 1994. *ERIC Digest*. Educational Resource Information Center. USA.)

References and Further Readings

1. Brookfield S. Adult Learning: An Overview. In: A. Tuinjman (ed.) 1995. *International Encyclopedia of Education*. Pergamon Press. Oxford. UK. (Accessed through Internet).
2. Knowles MS. Introduction: The Art and Science of Helping Adults Learn. In: *Andragogy in Action: Applying Modern Principles of Adult Learning*. 1984. Knowles MS *et al.* Jossey-Bass. San Francisco, California. USA.
3. Kopp K. Evaluate the Performance of Adults. Module N-6 of Category N. ERIC Document Reproduction Service No. ED 289969.
4. Imel S. Guidelines for Working with Adult Learners. 1994. *ERIC Digest*. No. 154. ERIC_NO: ED377313.
5. Lindeman ECL. 1926. The Meaning of Adult Education. New

Republic, New York. Quoted in 'Adult Learning: An Overview' by Stephen Brookfield in A. Tuinjman (ed.) (1995). *International Encyclopedia of Education*. Oxford, Pergamon Press. (Accessed through internet).

6. Rogers J. *Adults Learning*. Third Edition Philadelphia, PA: Open University Press, 1989.

7. Zemke R and Zemke S. 30 Things We Know for Sure About Adult Learning. University of Hawaii. Internet address: http://www.hcc.hawaii.edu/intranet/committees/FacDevCom /guidebk/teachtip/adults-3.htm. Accessed May 02.

5 Building the Skills of Learning

From the discussion of the earlier chapters, we recognize that the *skill of learning is a critical determinant of success of learning in learner-centered learning model*. In formal educational terminology, the skill of learning is known as metacognition.

In this chapter, our tasks are to

- Discuss the concepts of skills of learning
- Recognize the importance of the skills in learner-centered learning model
- Propose ways on how the skills can be instilled among the students

Flavell first proposed the concepts of skill of learning or metacognition in the seventies. Since then metacognition has become a significant feature of intelligence. Admittedly, the term is not in the common vocabulary of medical education partly because of the long and abstract nature of the word. But the concept is really simple. It is the knowledge of our own cognitive functions and the thinking about our own thinking process. In other words, this is the skill of learning how to learn.

Concepts of Metacognition

According to Flavell, metacognition includes *knowledge* and *regulation* about the process. Metacognition refers to our acquired knowledge about own cognitive ability and how such ability can be applied to the cognitive process. Further expansion of the theme suggests metacognition is related to person, task, and strategy. He identified these as 'variables' that determine the learning skills (Flavell, 79). Metacognitive skills are believed to be higher order cognitive skills that are necessary for the management of knowledge and other cognitive attributes.

Importance of Metacognition

Newer learning models delegate considerable importance of learning to the learners. The learners are required to set their own learning goals and execute appropriate learning methods to achieve the goals. The learners' responsibility also includes monitoring the progress of learning and alters the strategies whenever necessary. The empowerment of the learners to carry out their own learning is the cardinal feature of many models of learning including learner-centered learning, self-directed learning, and adult learning. A major determinant of success in such situations is the development of the ability and skills in learning.

Metacognition is also believed to be closely associated with intelligence. The learners who are better managers of their metacognitive skills are judged to be more intelligent and they are more likely to be successful than their peers who do not have the skills. Furthermore, direct instruction on metacognition is believed to improve learning among students (Scruggs, 1985).

Helping Students Develop Metacognitive Skills

What advice should we give to our students to be a skilled learner? How do we instill a metacognitive culture among our students?

For an individual learner, metacognition consist of the three basic simple steps very much analogous to the 'Learning Cycle' that we will discuss in the subsequent chapters. The basic steps are

- Identifying the needs
- Developing and implementing a plan of learning
- Monitoring and evaluating the progress

Identifying the needs

The first step is the exact determination of the current situation of an individual learner. The ideas are to identify the 'knowledge gap' or 'learning gap' and to help decide the priority areas that need to be addressed. The simple questions that help the learner in this step are

- What do I already know about the topic?
- What do I not know about the topic?
- What is the knowledge gap?
- What is the most important topic that I need to address?

Developing and implementing a plan of learning

In this stage, a plan for the learning is developed based on the known learning needs. The learning strategies are varied and unique to each individual learner. The learning strategy that is successful with one learner may not be so with other learners. The sample basic questions that need to be answered at this stage are:

- What learning strategy is most likely help me achieve the target?
- What alternative do I have?
- Is it the best strategy?
- What are the resources I need?
- Do I have prior success with this strategy?
- What is the type of monitoring and evaluation most suitable for this particular strategy?

Monitoring and evaluating the progress

Monitoring and evaluation of the progress is a continuous process. This step goes beyond simple collection of data about the progress. This also requires utilization of the data to amend and alter the learning strategy. The basic questions at this stage are

- What is the progress so far?
- Is the time frame realistic?
- Do I need to change the learning strategy?
- What is the most important determinant of my success or failure?
- What have I learned from the process that would help me in future?

Institution-wide implementation of metacognitive skills is also possible with deliberate and conscious effort by the teachers. The idea is to create a culture where such skills are expected and practiced.

Blakey and Spence (1990) suggested six basic strategies that are to be implemented by the teachers to develop metacongnitive behaviors in the students. These are

- Conscious identification of what students *"know"* as opposed to "what they don't know"
- Development of a *thinking vocabulary* so that the students can verbally describe their thinking processes
- Creation of a thinking journal or *learning log* for students to reflect upon their learning processes
- Assumption of *responsibility for regulating own learning activities*, including time requirements and organization of materials
- Ability to *review and evaluate* these strategies as either successful or inappropriate, and
- Participation in a *guided self-evaluation* through individual conferences and checklists focusing on the thinking process

Learning to learn is an emerging concept in education. As we advance towards implementation of learner-centered and other active and self-directed learning models, the skills of learning become even more important.

In summary, the important concepts that we have learned in this chapter are

- Metacognition is the skill of learning
- The skill of learning is an important element of learner-centered learning
- At individual learner level, the steps to promote metacognition include helping learner identify the educational needs, developing and implementing a plan, and monitoring and evaluation of the progress

References and Further Readings

1. Blakey E, and Spence S. Developing Metacognition. November 1990. ERIC Clearinghouse on Information Resources Syracuse NY. ERIC Identifier: ED 327218.
2. Flavell JH. Metacognition and Cognitive Monitoring: A New Area of Cognitive-Developmental Inquiry. *American Psychologist*. 1979. 34; 906–11.
3. Scruggs TE, Mastropieri MA, Monson J, and Jorgenson C. Maximizing What Gifted Students Can Learn: Recent Findings of Learning Strategy Research. *Gifted Child Quarterly*. 1985. 29(4), 181–5. EJ 333 116. Quoted in Blakey, Elaine and Spence, Sheila. Developing Metacognition. November 1990. ERIC. Syracuse NY. ERIC Identifier: ED 327218.

Section 4

Curriculum and Learning Cycle

6 Curriculum Design and Implementation

Discussions on curriculum are often limited to who 'covers' what,
an approach more suited to barn painting than to education.

Timothy Goldsmith, Science, 2002

Curriculum is an integral component of academic experience in medical schools. The complexity surrounding the curricular planning and implementation demands that the supervision of the tasks be entrusted to the experts who have the necessary expertise and experience in this field. Nevertheless, individual medical teachers are intimately involved in the curriculum planning and implementation as well and they are frequently asked to serve as a member of the curriculum committee.

In this chapter, our tasks are to

- Define curriculum in the light of prevalent and contemporary educational theories
- Discuss the basic steps in curricular planning and implementation
- Elaborate the systematic approach to curriculum planning and implementation

- Discuss the barriers to curricular innovations and ways to overcome them

Definition

Definitions of curriculum are abundant. Unfortunately, the plethora of definition also creates confusion and misunderstanding. Therefore, we have adopted a simplified and practical approach in defining the curriculum. Essentially our approach is to view the curriculum as an academic plan that is made up of several steps that also explain the roles and functions of a curriculum. This approach to curricular definition seems to be the most relevant because, in addition to the concept, it also states clearly and concretely the practical steps to take.

To begin with it is important to be aware of what is *not* a curriculum so as not to be confused. A curriculum is not a syllabus, a timetable of lectures, or a listing of lectures by discipline. Similarly, curriculum is not a teaching program written by clinicians or basic scientists based on their own expertise and interest. A teaching program without room provided for feedback from peers and students for revision does not qualify to be a curriculum.

Thus, a curriculum, defined as an academic plan or total experience, suggests that *curriculum design and implementation should follow a series of steps that operates like a spiral that goes both upwards and downwards with a feedback system for adjustment at every step*. This approach is similar to the 'educational spiral' or 'learning cycle' which has been proposed and implemented in health professional training (Guilbert, 1981) that also highlights the importance of systematic and sequential progression of goal settings, implementation, evaluation, and modification.

In general, curriculum, as an academic plan, contains several key elements that include the goals of the program, content to be taught and learned, the sequence of implementation, the teaching strategies to achieve the goals, description and allocation of resources, and a detailed plan for evaluation and adjustment (Stark,

1997). Among a multitude of existing curriculum models, the Johns Hopkins University Medical School adopted a six-step approach to academic planning to address the design and implementation of a medical curriculum (Table 1) (Kern *et al*, 1998). This curricular model is based on learner-centered learning strategies and emphasizes proper consideration of the profiles of the target, namely the students.

Step one: Identification of the faculty/institution's mission and the needs of its stakeholders

The crucial first step in curriculum design is to formulate a mission statement of the medical school. Frequently such mission statements are already in existence but need necessary updating. The mission statement of a school of medicine is largely determined by societal and national health care needs and priorities and aspiration. The mission of a faculty of medicine is to train doctors to deliver effective health care services based on these factors. Consequently, the mission statement of medical schools varies considerably and it is strongly recommended that each medical school develops mission statements of its own.

As the mission statements of the medical school are reflective of larger societal and national needs, there are many stakeholders with substantial interest in determining the profile of medical graduates. The range of stakeholders may include students, faculty members, university administrators, professional and regulatory bodies, and the government. Faculty members involved in curriculum planning must be cognizant of these diverse groups of stakeholders and be appropriately sensitive to their needs and recommendations.

In the late nineties, The Faculty of Medicine, National University of Singapore embarked on a curricular reform process to realign the faculty's mission. It also decided on the gradual adaptation of newer paradigms in medical education. The reform process resulted in the creation of new mission statements that emphasizes, in addition to the ability to practice medicine in a sound and effective manner, other qualities such as critical analytical ability, self-directed and life-long learning, good communication skills, and compassion and ethical standard.

To achieve these missions, the medical curriculum was also re-designed. One of the elements was the creation of two main components in the curriculum: the core and the special study modules (SSM). Inclusion of the SSM was based on the realization that a certain degree of flexibility and independence is necessary for the students to master the newer and broader missions. Therefore, the core curriculum covered that part of the curriculum that all students should study and master, while the SSM provided students with an option to study an area in depth (Harden, 2001). The SSM also includes, in addition to pure medical subjects, other non-medical and para-medical topics such as art, history, and social sciences.

Step two: Needs assessment of the learners

The second step in curricular planning involves comprehensive needs assessment of the learners including learners' strengths and weaknesses in order to develop more appropriate instructional methods and assessment instruments.

The following are examples of needs assessment data that are relevant for curriculum planning and implementation:

- Entry level of competence
- Prior educational experience
- Exposure and success with self-directed and group study
- Ability to meet the requirements of the program
- Individual goals and priorities
- Personal background including reasons for enrolling
- Attitudes towards the discipline
- Assumptions and expectations from the program

Step three: Establishment of the curriculum's goals and objectives

Goals and objectives determine the instructional philosophy and thus guide the selection of the most effective learning methods. Moreover, learning objectives are crucial for the design and selection of assessment instruments and procedures. Clear and well-written objectives communicate the focus of the medical curriculum to all stakeholders. It also ensures that the ultimate educational experiences of the learners are in line with the faculty's mission statements.

Curricular goals should be set according to the three domains of education: knowledge, skills, and attitudes (Hendrie & Lloyd, 1990). Curricular goals should also take into account newer trends and evidence-based practices in medical education such as *reduction* of factual information, active learning, vertical and horizontal integration of subjects, early clinical exposure, and balance between hospital and community-based medicine (Towle in Joly and Rees, 1998).

Step four: Selection of educational strategies

The selection of educational strategies is based on three cardinal principles. First, the educational strategy or instructional methods must be congruent with the learning objectives. Thus, a program objective that emphasizes the development of competency in interviewing skills must have a structured instructional method that includes interview with real or simulated patients. Other forms of instructional strategy such as lecture and paper and pencil case, although important, are not sufficient without the actual practice of interview.

Second, the use of multiple instructional strategies is preferable to a single method and will be more likely to meet the demands of the specific learning situations. Curriculum should be responsive and flexible enough to take into account the diversity and individuality of the students including their preferred learning style. Finally, the curriculum designer and implementer must verify the curriculum's feasibility in terms of material and human resources.

Step five: Assessment of students

Education is a process that brings changes in student behavior. If a desirable behavior does not take place, the curriculum is largely considered a failure. Therefore, student assessment is one of the measures of the intended behavior change that the curriculum is entrusted to achieve.

Student assessment is of paramount importance in curriculum planning. Assessment instruments need to be carefully pre-selected and planned so that they meet the requisite reliability and validity for the purpose. Despite efforts of medical educators to put emphasis on learning objectives as the driving force in a curriculum, a good and congruent examination system is equally important as the student's dedication to study is often triggered by this last factor. It is strongly recommended that the student assessment be planned at the inception alongside with setting of the learning objectives and never left to be decided at the end.

Step six: Evaluation and monitoring of the curriculum

Although evaluation of the curriculum is the last step in this practical approach, it is not necessarily the final action. The evaluation data collected serve as a criteria for adjusting the curriculum according to the goals of the program or the mission of the faculty. Importantly, it also convinces and reassures the faculty members about the effectiveness of the new curriculum.

The most important message is that a curriculum is a *dynamic* process. It must be evaluated, corrected, monitored and gone through repeated levels of innovation and adjustment. Collection of feedback from teachers, tutors and students must be ongoing. The feedback should be given appropriate and serious consideration and the results should be communicated back to the faculty members.

We realize that curriculum planning and implementation is a detailed exercise that progresses sequentially with continuing monitoring and modifications. As such, design and implementation of curriculum can be long. The planning phase of the curriculum may take up to two years. Depending upon the preparedness and commitment of the faculty members and medical schools, the implementation phase may require three to five years (Kantrowitz *et al*, 1987).

A curriculum is an academic plan. It is a total blueprint for action where

- The objectives, aims and outcomes of the curriculum are clarified
- The processes to achieve these are identified
- A careful evaluation plan about the success in pre-defined
- Systematic review and adjustment are regularly implemented

Strategies for Implementation of Curriculum Innovations

Recommendations for reform in medical education abound. The barriers to such reform are not a lack of educational imagination but a lack of skills in clearly diagnosing the barriers to institutional change and skills in mounting an effective strategy for overcoming institutional inertia.

Stewart P Mennin and Arthur Kaufman, 1989

Historically, any change attempt in medical education has been viewed with incredible suspicion and many were aborted prematurely due to outright rejection. Such resistance to change is almost universal and witnessed in medical schools undergoing reform process. In most cases such innovations failed to come into reality not because of the lack of robustness in the innovations but rather from the inability of curricular planners to anticipate and plan properly for the source of the resistance.

The resistance to change may come from many fronts. Potentially, every stakeholder in the curriculum may oppose curricular reform for a variety of reasons. Experience from the medical schools with major reform initiatives frequently points out that the major resistance originates in the faculty members (Mennin and Kaufman, 1989). The resistance from faculty members is especially viewed with trepidation by the curricular reformers as the actual implementation of the curriculum heavily depends on their buy-in and active participation.

One of the most important reasons for the faculty members to resist any curricular change is the *fear of loss of control*. A medical school is like a complex social organization with many competing departments and institutions (Bloom, 1989). During reform initiatives each department and individuals within the department often tends to become territorial with the tendency to keep control over their own turf. These usually translate into keeping check on the content coverage, methods of teaching, and assessment processes. In other words, every department tends to decide what is to be taught, how much, what way, when, and by whom.

Fortunately and interestingly enough, this pattern of response is rather *generic* and tends to take place all over the world (Mennin and Kaufman, 1989). There is a remarkable degree of consistency and similarity in the pattern for resistance despite the cultural, sociological, and organizational differences in medical schools. Thus, it is possible to predict these resistances in advance and prepare the reform process accordingly.

Mennin and Kaufman in their seminal treatise on the change process suggested several strategies to facilitate reform process. The importance of creation of broad-based ownership is indisputable. Curricular reform is unlikely to be successfully carried out by a handful of selected individuals. Rather, a multidisciplinary team made up of clinicians and basic scientists from different disciplines provides a dependable foundation of expertise that would propagate the reform process.

Such a multidisciplinary team approach to curricular design serves several critical functions. By bringing people from different backgrounds, the team members learn to interact with each other and form a strong and coherent group that plays a crucial role at the implementation phase of that curriculum. Strategically, early involvement of the faculty members guarantees the necessary commitment and the participation of members in the project. The faculty members are more likely to accept the new curriculum if their opinions are *proactively and prospectively sought, valued, and incorporated.*

Besides the faculty members, the students are another major group with substantial stakes in the curriculum. They are the most immediate 'consumer' of medical education and all the curricular initiatives are directed towards them. The chance of success in the curricular reform greatly improves with active support from the students. Faculty members are more likely to be receptive of curricular innovation if the students voice their support for the new curriculum. The presence of a vibrant student group that actively advocates, and rallies support for the new curriculum can have a catalytic effect on the reform process.

The experience from the University of Airlangga, Indonesia speaks favorably about the beneficial effect of students on curricular innovation. Recently, the university decided to implement problem-based learning in medical school. During the early phase of implementation, the university decided to send a selected group of medical students to neighboring Singapore where PBL has been successfully implemented for some time. The visiting students participated in the educational activities and received first-hand experience on the PBL process. After returning to their home institute they have become the most vocal proponent for change. The faculty members, who were incredulous and reluctant, are more receptive to PBL now.

The tasks of curricular design are also boosted by the active presence of faculty members with background in medical education or experience in curriculum planning. Curriculum design, innovation, and changes are continuously practiced in many medical schools with genuine interest in implementing an excellent program to train future doctors. The experience from such medical schools is a valuable resource during curricular planning and implementation and should be sought as well.

Strategies for Curricular Reform
(Mennin and Kaufman, 1989)

- Building a broad-base ownership for change
- Test and modify innovations frequently
- Develop understanding through participation
- Demonstrate ability to compromise
- Describe new program as experiment
- Share rewards

Finally, a strong leadership with a clear vision provided by the dean of the medical school is an essential prerequisite to advocate the necessity for changes in the existing curriculum. The dean can greatly facilitate the implementation process by way of explaining the relevance of changes and innovation in the new curriculum.

The Chinese character for 'change' has dual connotations to it: on the one hand it means 'danger', on the other hand it also means 'opportunity.' During a change in an educational organization it is up to the initiator of the change process to determine whether the change would turn out to be an opportunity or a danger. With clear understandings of the underlying principles of curriculum and proper planning of the change during curricular reform, it is more likely to be an opportunity for the medical teachers to create a nurturing and supportive learning environment.

In summary, the most important points that we have learned are

- Curriculum is a dynamic process that needs a systemic and stepwise implementation
- Curriculum should have a built-in feedback system with ample room for ongoing modification and adjustment
- Every curricular reform faces a predictable pattern of resistance

- A broad-based consensus among the faculty members is crucial for successful implementation
- Support from the dean and the students has very valuable impact on the reform process

References and Further Readings

1. Bloom SW. The Medical School as a Social Organization: The Sources of Resistance to Change. *Medical Education*. 1989. 23: 228–41.
2. Brian J, and Lesley R. *Medical Education in the Millennium*. Oxford, Oxford University Press, 1998.
3. Dent JA, and Harden R. *A Practical Guide for Medical Teachers*. Edinburgh, Churchill Livingston, 2001.
4. Goldsmith T. 2002. *Science*. 297: 1769.
5. Guilbert J-J. *Educational Handbook for Health Personnel*. Geneva. World Health Organization. 1981.
6. Hendrie HC, and Lloyd C. Educating Competent and Humane Physicians. Indianapolis, Indiana University Press. USA. 1990.
7. Kantrowitz M, Kaufman A, Mennin S, Fulop T, and Guilbert J-J (editors). *Innovative Tracks in the Established Institutions for the Education of Health Personnel*. 1987. WHO Offset Publication Number 11. WHO. Geneva. Switzerland.
8. Kern DE, Thomas PA, Howard DM, and Bass EB. *Curriculum Development for Medical Education*. Baltimore. The Johns Hopkins University Press, 1998.
9. Mennin SP, and Kaufmann A. The Change Process and Medical Education. *Medical Teacher*. 1989. 11(1): 39–46.
10. Stark JS. *Shaping the College Curriculum: Academic Plans in Action*. Boston. Allyn and Bacon. 1997.

7 Learning Cycle

The design of an educational program—be it curriculum or a course—is based on three essential elements: (a) learning objectives, (b) instructional methodology, and (c) assessment and evaluation. These three elements form the foundation on which the entire educational program is structured. The three elements are variously described as 'educational spiral' or 'learning cycle' (Guilbert, 1981).

The learning objectives convey the purpose of educational program. They succinctly and clearly describe what are to be learned from the educational program. Instructional methods elaborate the best possible way to achieve the learning objectives. The assessment process monitors the progress of the educational activities and determines whether the objectives of the program have been reached. Information from the assessment should feedback into the cycle for further refinement and readjustment.

Let us use an analogy to describe the process. If we are to plan a trip, the destination that we want to reach would be our objectives of the travel. This would be described by the question 'Where do we want to go?' A parallel question in educational planning would be 'What do we want our learners to learn?' Once the destination

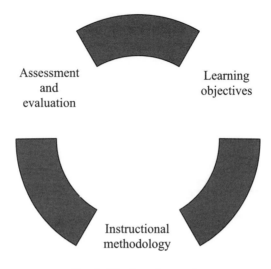

Fig. 1. The learning cycle.

is decided upon, the next decision point is to decide on the mode of the journey as exemplified by the question 'How do we want to travel to the destination?' A parallel question is educational planning would be 'How do we want the learners to learn to achieve the objectives?' Once these have been decided upon, the next two important questions pertain to whether we have reached the destination and questions in this respect are 'Have we reached the destination?' and 'What have we learned from the journey?' The answer from the last question would also help us better prepare for the next journey. The analogous questions in educational planning would be 'Have we met the learning objectives?' and 'How can we further improve the education program?'

Although many suggest a linear relationship between the three components—objective is the first step, then the method, and finally the assessment, an alternate and perhaps more logical way of understanding the relationship between the three is that objectives, instructional methods, and assessment are intertwined and rarely separable from each other.

The concept of inter-dependency deserves further elaboration. Firstly, the three elements of the learning cycles are *inter-related and constitute three pillars* on which the entire educational program is structured. Weakening of any one component results in weakening of the entire structure and makes the program vulnerable to failure. Thus, good educational objectives alone without matching instructional methods and congruous assessment system are unlikely to bring any meaningful result from the educational program. Similarly, a weakened instructional method, even if supported by good learning objectives and assessment, corrodes the very basic foundation and is unlikely to succeed.

Secondly, the chance of success of the educational program improves if the three elements are determined and planned from *the very inception of the program*. Early planning provides an opportunity for medical educators to think thoroughly and prospectively about all aspects of educational activities. As these three elements are inter-related and coupled with each other, early planning is vital for keeping the three components in synergy.

We follow the theme of learning cycle in the organization of the subsequent chapters. Thus, first we describe the learning objectives, including ways to write them. Subsequently, we progress to instructional methods such as lectures, small group, and role-play. Included here are clinical teaching and problem-based learning as well. Finally, we describe various aspects of student assessment.

Reference and Further Reading

1. Guilbert J-J. *Educational Handbook for Health Personnel*. Geneva. World Health Organization. 1981.

Section 5

Educational Objectives

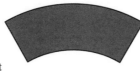

Assessment
and
evaluation

**Educational
objectives**

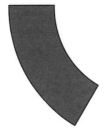

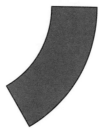

Instructional
methodology

8 Classification of Educational Objectives

The first step of educational planning involves deciding and conveying the objectives of the educational program in a systematic manner. Educational objectives are generally structured around several classification systems known as *taxonomies of educational objectives*. Among these, the most commonly used classification system is Bloom's taxonomy.

In this chapter, we follow Bloom's proposed classification system and

- Describe and analyze three broad categories or domains of educational objectives
- Separate and sub-classify these domains into a hierarchical pattern
- Review examples of educational objectives within each domain and their sub-classification

Education is a broad umbrella term that encompasses many complex and interconnected activities. In 1956, Benjamin Bloom and his co-workers attempted to classify educational activities based on the *objectives of education*. They proposed that such objectives fall into three broad categories or domains: (a) cognitive or knowledge, (b) psychomotor or skills, and (c) affective or attitudes. This classification provides a useful structure and determines the level of sophistication expected from the learners. Because assessment and evaluation is directly linked to educational objectives, Bloom's classification is also used extensively in assessment and evaluation. Another added advantage of Bloom's classification system, pertinent to medical science, is that this classification conforms to the American Psychological Association's recommendations and is commonly used in various psychometric testings.

Each of three broad domains of education (knowledge, skill, and attitudes) is further sub-classified into a hierarchical pattern known as *levels*. The higher levels in this hierarchy are more complex and intellectually demanding than the lower levels. Generally, objectives at the lower levels are mastered first before higher level objectives are accomplished and the learners sequentially progress from one level to the next. For example, typically the learners need to attain certain factual 'knowledge' about a topic before being able to understand the underlying concepts. And, once they 'understand' the concepts well they are able to utilize or 'apply' the concepts into practice. Thus, knowledge leads to understanding and understanding in turn is necessary for application.

Educational Objectives

↓

Domains

↓

Levels

Research and experience have shown that we, as medical teachers, tend to confine ourselves to a certain level within a domain and conduct our educational activities from that level only. Most of the time, this comfort zone represents lower levels of educational objectives. There is reluctance and resistance towards using higher levels during educational activities such as objective settings, questioning, as well as during student assessment and evaluation. Much of this reluctance results from unfamiliarity with this classification system and perhaps also due to abstract sounding terminology associated with it. In reality, the basic structure and logic in this classification system are fairly simple and straightforward. Familiarity with this classification system is crucial to overcome the psychological and technical barriers and to help us construct meaningful educational objectives.

Table 1. Understanding Bloom's proposed classification system.

Bloom's Proposed Terms	What is it?	Examples	Substitution of the Terms
Cognitive Domain	• Knowledge • Intellect	• Decision making • Understanding a concept	Knowledge
Psychomotor Domain	• Manual dexterity • Physical skills	• Ability to operate equipment • Laceration repair	Skills
Affective Domain	• Behavior • Attitudes	• Empathy towards patients • Respect for individual	Attitudes

One fine morning, I decided to learn driving a car. I realized that learning to drive a car is a constellation of several learning activities. First, I need to recognize and interpret the road signs. This is knowledge (cognition). Second, I need to maneuver the car properly and keep it on track. This is skill (psychomotor). Finally, I need to develop some road manners and courtesy for my fellow drivers. This is attitude (affective). Thus, driving a car is an educational or learning activity that comprises knowledge, skills, and attitude.

Cognitive Domain

The cognitive domain is demonstrated by knowledge recall and intellectual skills. The preliminary levels in cognitive domain are simple knowledge acquisition and utilization of memory. Subsequently, these progress towards understanding and comprehension of the meaning of the newly acquired information. The next level involves application of the knowledge. Higher levels require increasingly more complex mental processes and include analysis, synthesis, and evaluation. Some educators associate the last three levels of cognitive domain with problem solving.

In the subsequent sections, we will explore the various levels within the cognitive domain. We will use a real teaching encounter as an example to determine the educational objectives for each level.

Clinical Scenario: You are conducting ward round with your medical officers in the Neonatal Intensive Care Unit. The patient JK is an extremely premature baby with chronic lung disease. One of the medical officers proposes dexamethasone (a steroid) therapy for JK. Although dexamethasone improves lung function in chronic lung disease, you are aware of many side effects of such therapy. Specifically, you are concerned about several recent reports of adverse neurological outcomes that are associated with prolonged dexamethasone therapy. You want to promote critical thinking in your medical officers and decide to seize upon this opportunity.

The six levels of cognitive ladder in Bloom's Taxonomy, from lower level to higher level, are: (1) knowledge, (2) comprehension, (3) application, (4) analysis, (5) synthesis, and (6) evaluation (Fig. 1).

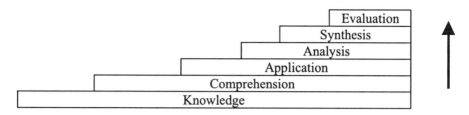

Fig. 1. The cognitive ladder. (From Bloom, 1956)

Level one: Knowledge

Knowledge is the ability to recall or remember previously learned materials without much understanding of the meaning. Examples of knowledge level include ability to recall specific facts or common terms and identify part of a diagram.

- Representative verbs: list, write, identify
- Illustration of objective: Medical officers will be able to list at least eight side effects of dexamethasone therapy in premature infants.

Level two: Comprehension

Comprehension follows acquisition of knowledge by the learners. It is exemplified by the ability to understand the meaning of an idea or a concept.

- Representative verbs: differentiate between, discriminate, interpret
- Illustration of objective: Medical officers will be able to explain the mechanisms of weight loss during dexamethasone therapy.

Level three: Application

In the application level, the learner shows ability to use or apply the learned concepts and ideas. Examples of these include application of principles in new situations and demonstration of correct use of procedures.

- Representative verbs: apply, demonstrate, operate
- Illustration of objective: When provided with given formula to calculate body surface area and a drug dosage handbook, medical officers will be able to determine the correct dexamethasone dosage regimen for a particular patient.

Level four: Analysis

Analysis is the ability to separate a complex concept into component parts and establish relationship between the parts. Examples include ability to determine the relevance and usefulness of information and correlate between the information.

- Representative verbs: analyze, categorize, diagnose, outline
- Illustration of objective: Medical officers will be able to outline the components of a care plan to monitor for the anticipated side effects of dexamethasone therapy.

Level five: Synthesis

Synthesis involves construction of new ideas or hypotheses and establishment of new relationship between the theories. Examples of synthesis include ability to write a well-organized theme, write a research proposal, and plan an experiment.

- Representative verbs: construct, synthesize, propose
- Illustration of objective: Medical officers will be able to propose a hypothesis that will explain the possible mechanism of adverse neurological outcomes that are associated with prolonged dexamethasone usage.

Level six: Evaluation

According to Bloom's classification, evaluation is the highest level of cognitive domain and is demonstrated by the ability to judge the worth of data against stated criteria. Evaluation level examples include ability to judge the value of a research paper, compare between treatment modalities, and select appropriate treatment guideline for own patient population.

- Representative verbs: judge, compare, validate
- Illustration of objective: Using a set of criteria, medical officers will be able to rank the research papers on dexamethasone therapy according to the strength of their evidence.

Psychomotor Domain

Psychomotor domain is demonstrated by physical skills such as co-ordination, dexterity, manipulation, strength, and speed. Examples of common psychomotor domain in clinical medicine include setting an intravenous drip, airway intubation, and laceration repairs.

Psychomotor domain is therefore a combination of 'psycho' (knowledge, cognition) and motor skills. In medicine, psychomotor domain has a strong 'psycho' or knowledge component. For example, although airway intubation is a psychomotor skill, the learners require significant background knowledge of upper airway anatomy and disease processes before being able to perform the procedure.

Psychomotor learning is sequential and learners generally acquire the skills in the following order:

Imitation

This is the earliest level of learning a complex skill. At the beginning, the learner indicates his readiness to experiment with the skill and reacts by imitating the skill that has been demonstrated or explained to him.

Manipulation

In this level, the individual learner continues to practice the particular skill or the sequence until it becomes his own habit and the action can be performed with some degree of confidence and proficiency.

Precision

Skill is attained at this level and demonstrated by a quick, smooth, accurate performance that requires minimum energy and effort by the learner.

Articulation

The skills are well developed at this stage and the learner confidently modifies movement patterns to fit special requirements or to meet a problem situation.

Naturalization

This is the final level of psychomotor learning. The skill is characterized by natural and effortless automatism. The learner demonstrates the naturalization by way of experiments or discovering new motor acts by manipulating the materials based on an understanding of how they work.

Affective Domain

Affective learning is demonstrated by behaviors that indicate attitude of awareness, interest, attention, concern, responsibility, and ability to listen and respond during interactions with others. Examples of affective learning include the ability to express empathy with the patients and respecting the patients' privacy and confidentiality. This is the domain that is often, albeit in narrow sense, associated with the meaning of 'professionalism' in medicine. This domain relates to emotions, attitudes, appreciation, and values and is expressed in a variety of ways such as enjoyment, respect, and support. As these qualities are subjective and closely associated with individual judgements and morality, affective domain is inherently difficult to evaluate.

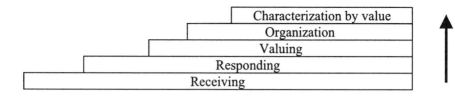

Fig. 2. The levels of affective domain. (From Krathwohl, Bloom, and Masia, 1956).

Krathwohl, Bloom, and Masia proposed progressive levels of learning and incorporation of affective domains that are somewhat analogous to cognitive ladder (Fig. 2).

We will use a real teaching scenario to illustrate how the affective domain can be applied to everyday teaching.

> Teaching Scenario: You are conducting a session with the nursing personnel to improve medication safety and to reduce medication errors. Your aim is to inculcate high professional values and eventual incorporation of certain behavior changes in your staff that will lead to reduction of medication errors.

Receiving

This is often the first level in affective learning where the learner is aware of something learnable in the environment. At this level, the learner may listen to a lecture or presentation about the safety models but she may or may not accept it.

- Illustration of objective: The learner will listen attentively to the presentation about medication safety.

Responding

The learner is more aware and responds to the lecture or the presentation. Such awareness or responsiveness is manifested by various actions of the learner such as answering questions, raising issues related to the topic, or attentively writing lecture notes.

- Illustration of objective: The learner will demonstrate her response by asking questions about the safety models.

Valuing

The learner shows some definite involvement or commitment. This commitment may be demonstrated by discussing the issue with fellow colleagues, urging others to attend the course, and advancing her education by incorporating some concepts from the presentation.

- Illustration of objective: The learner will encourage her colleagues to learn and to make use of safety models in the prevention of medication errors.

Organization

The learner integrates the new value into her general set of values by ranking it among her general priorities. This is the level at which the learner organizes herself in making long-term commitments to the newly learned model and incorporates the model into her own practice.

- Illustration of objective: The learner will apply the new safety model into her practice.

Characterization by value

The learner champions the new value and consistently acts according to the newly incorporated value. This is the highest level of affective learning that is demonstrated by firm commitment and willingness to advance the value. The learner becomes the role model for others and organizes instructions or champions the newly learned values.

- Illustration of objective: The learner will organize medication safety courses for her colleagues on her own initiative.

Table 2. Examples of verbs in cognitive domain. Note some of the verbs are used in more than one level (Bloom, 1956).

Knowledge	Comprehension	Application	Analysis	Synthesis	Evaluation
Define	Choose	Apply	Analyze	Assemble	Appraise
Identify	Cite examples of	Demonstrate	Categorize	Compose	Assess
List	Describe	Generalize	Compare	Construct	Choose
Name	Determine	Illustrate	Conclude	Create	Compare
Recall	Discriminate	Interpret	Contrast	Design	Critique
Recognize	Discuss	Operate	Correlate	Develop	Estimate
Record	Explain	Practice	Criticize	Formulate	Evaluate
Repeat	Identify	Relate	Debate	Organize	Judge
Underline	Interpret	Use	Detect	Plan	Measure
	Restate	Utilize	Determine	Prepare	Rate
	Review	Initiate	Develop	Produce	Revise
	Recognize		Differentiate	Propose	Score
	Tell		Examine	Predict	Select
	Simulates		Experiment	Reconstruct	Validate
			Infer	Set-up	Value
			Predict	Synthesize	Test
			Question	Devise	
			Relate		
			Solve		
			Test		
			Diagnose		

Table 3. Verbs applicable to psychomotor and affective domain. (Krathwohl, Bloom, and Masia, 1956).

Psychomotor	Affective domain
Bend, grasp, handle, operate, reach, relax, shorten, stretch, write, differentiate (by touch), express (facially), perform (skillfully)	Accepts, attempts, challenges, judges, defends, disputes, joins, praises, questions, shares, supports, and volunteers

Tables 2 and 3 list some of the verbs that are commonly used to describe cognitive, psychomotor, and affective domains. We can use these verbs to write educational objectives and to formulate questions during teaching. These verbs are used for educational assessment and evaluation as well. In the next chapter, we will discuss how to use the framework of Blooms' classification system to write educational objectives.

In summary, in this chapter, we have learned

- Educational objectives are divided into three somewhat overlapping broad domains: cognitive (knowledge), psychomotor (skills), and affective (attitudes)
- Each of these domains are sub-classified into different levels that follow a hierarchical pattern
- The classification system is useful for many commonly performed educational activities such as developing learning objective, questioning during teaching, and assessment

References and Further Readings

1. Bloom BS. (Ed.) *Taxonomy of Educational Objectives: The Classification of Educational Goals: Handbook I, Cognitive Domain.* 1956. Toronto: Longmans, Green: New York. USA.
2. Guilbert J-J. *Educational Handbook for Health Personnel.* 1981. World Health Organization. Geneva.
3. Krathwohl D, Bloom B, and Masia B. *Taxonomy of Educational Objectives. Handbook II: Affective Domain.* 1956. David McKay. New York. USA.

"Cheshire Puss," said Alice, "would you tell me, please, which way I ought to walk from here?"
"That depends a good deal on where you want to get to," said the Cat.
"I don't much care where," said Alice.
"Then it doesn't matter which way you walk," said the Cat.

"–so long as I get *somewhere*," Alice added as an explanation. "Oh, you're sure to do that," said the Cat, "if you only walk long enough."

(Carroll, Alice in Wonderland. As quoted in Health Care Education: A Guide to Staff Development. By Barbara K. Parker. Appleton-Century-Crofts. Norwalk, CT, USA)

9 Writing Educational Objectives

If you are not certain of where you are going you may very well end-up somewhere else (and not even know it).

Mager

In the earlier chapter, we have learned about Bloom's proposed classification system and other fundamental aspects of educational objectives. In this chapter, we will learn how to write good educational objectives that would convey our intentions in a meaningful way.

Thus, in this chapter, our tasks are to

- Discuss the purposes of educational objectives
- Identify their components and characteristics
- Construct educational objectives to meet our own teaching needs

Educational objectives are short, well-structured statements that specify what the learners are expected to achieve at the end of an educational program. They usually contain descriptions of *specific*, *short-term*, *measurable*, and *observable* behaviors that the program intends to achieve in the learners. A related term, educational goal, on the other hand is somewhat broad, generalized statements about the overall purpose of the program. Educational objectives are often referred to as *learning objectives* to emphasize that educational objectives describe what the 'learners' should be able to achieve as opposed to what the teachers want to teach.

The Purpose of Educational Objectives

As we have learned from earlier chapters, the three essential components of educational planning are (a) objectives, (b) instructional methods, and (c) assessment and evaluation. Together they form the foundation upon which the structure of an educational program is built. Weakening of any one of the components is likely to jeopardize the educational program as a whole. As we move towards writing good educational objectives it is essential that we constantly remind ourselves of this relationship and the interdependence between these three elements.

Good educational objectives benefit both the teachers and the learners. According to Paul Ramsden (1992), the most compelling reason for using aims and objectives is to *explain the intentions of the teachers to the learners*. He argued that at the beginning of any educational program there is uncertainty and confusion among the learners regarding the purpose of the program. Without a clear sense of direction they waste time and embark on many unproductive activities and are less likely to succeed. Finally, the lack of success contributes to a decline in motivation for attending the program. Good educational objectives help the learners to remain focused during the educational endeavor and minimize wastage of efforts and vastly improve their chance of success.

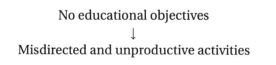

No educational objectives
↓
Misdirected and unproductive activities

↓
Lesser chance of success
↓
Unmotivated learners

While we tend to think, rightly so, that educational objectives benefit the learners, many fail to appreciate the benefits that the *teachers gain* too from good educational objectives. Teaching is a lot about self-reflection. It involves ongoing and deliberate assessment, reorganization, and planning of educational activities by the teachers. Ramsden again pointed out that we often do not pay adequate attention during planning of an educational program and tend to be reserved about self-reflection. The process of writing educational objectives demands that we, as teachers, critically and consciously reflect upon our teaching efforts and think about the learning activities and progress made by the learners. Thus, good educational objectives act as an impetus for the teachers to think prospectively about the program's effectiveness and ways to achieve the objectives from the very onset of the program.

Thus, the purposes of educational objectives are many

- To convey without ambiguity and with specificity what knowledge, skills, or attitudes and behavioral change the learners expect to gain from the program
- To clarify these items to ourselves as teachers
- To determine the appropriate instructional methods to achieve the target
- To serve as the baseline upon which the assessment will be based

Characteristics of Good Educational Objectives

As it has been discussed in the earlier sections, educational objectives are learner-centered and contain descriptions of what the learners will be able to achieve at the end of the program. These outcomes should be measurable or at least observable and expressed without ambiguity.

Learner-centered educational objectives focus on the learners' achievements from the educational program. Let us consider two contrasting statements: (a) 'The objective of this chapter is to teach the readers how to write good educational objectives' and (b) 'After reading this chapter, the reader will be able to explain the guidelines for writing good educational objectives.' The first statement conveys the objective of the writer. In contrast, the second statement emphasizes what the readers (learners) should be able to do at the end of reading this chapter and hence is more learner-centered.

Educational objectives also specify desired learning outcomes in the learners. The emphasis here is on the outcome and not on the activity that the learners embark on during the program. An example of measurable or observable outcome is 'Students will correctly *identify* four out of five anatomical structures of the heart as outlined in the figure.' In contrast, an example of non-measurable behavior is 'Students will *observe* the video depicting the dissection of the heart.' The term 'observe' is non-measurable and is therefore an example of a poor educational objective. The first example also highlights the degree of measure ('four out of five').

Educational objectives should be high in clarity and easy to understand. A statement like 'Students will know about the childhood vaccines' is faulty from the point of educational objectives. The statement fails to convey what the examiners really mean by 'know'. In contrast, a well-constructed educational objective is 'Students will correctly describe the routine childhood immunization schedules in Singapore.' Here it is easy for the learners to understand what they are expected to know. Also, it is easier to link the assessment with the last objectives.

There are certain verbs that need to be avoided in writing educational objectives. These unsuitable verbs convey vague messages and lack the specificity required for writing educational objectives. For example, an objective which state 'student will realize ...' is open to interpretation. Similarly, the term 'understand' communicates different meaning to different individual and doesn't specify

Table 1. Strong and weak verbs in cognitive domain.

Non-specific Verbs	Alternate Examples
Know	Identify
Understand	Describe
Appreciate	Evaluate
Encourage	Recognize
Realize	
Remember	

any particular action that needs to be taken by the learners. Verbs that also need to be avoided include: know, appreciate, and think.

Thus, good educational objectives are

- Learner-centered
- Specific in describing the learning outcomes
- Pertaining to measurable or observable behaviors
- High in clarity and understandability
- Directly linked to assessment

Components of Educational Objectives

Generally, educational objectives are written in a structured way. Four essential components of that structure are:

- Target audience: Who are the learners?
- Observable/measurable behavior: What do we expect the learners to achieve?
- Condition: What are the conditions? What are the prerequisites? How do the learners achieve their targets?
- Degree: What is the extent of achievement? How much should they learn? Is there a specific criterion that we want our learners to meet?

The mnemonic for these four components is ABCD (for Audience, Behavior, Condition, and Degree).

Let us consider these examples:

'At the end of the two-hour tutorial and using the illustration, first year medical students will correctly identify eight out of ten anatomical structures of the heart.' In this example, 'first year medical students' is the audience, 'identify' is the measurable behavior, 'using the illustration' is the condition, and 'eight out of ten' anatomical structures of the heart is the degree. This is also an example of educational objectives for knowledge domain. For the psychomotor domain, a parallel example may be 'At the end of this skill station, the house officer will be able to accurately measure blood pressure all the time using a right-cuff and right anatomical landmark.' In this example 'house officer' is the audience, 'measure' in the observable behavior, 'using a right-cuff and right anatomical landmark' is the condition, and 'all the time' is the degree.

As we move up along the 'cognitive ladder' in Bloom's classification, it may become more difficult to specify the degree or the extent by which educational objectives need to be met. Therefore, a certain degree of latitude is permissible and may be necessary in specifying the degree of the target with higher order cognitive objectives.

Pitfalls to Avoid

Frequently we try to write educational objectives that focus on measurable behavior only. This is more likely to happen when objectives are written for lower steps in the cognitive ladder. It is rather enticing to choose verbs such as list and quantify the outcome (for example: 'Participants will be able to list all five bones of the wrist.'). Although such objectives are relatively easy to write, these can potentially narrow down the content coverage and may inhibit the learners' desire to learn and explore.

We also tend to write objectives that describe the content that will be covered in the course without specifying the target outcome. It is not uncommon to encounter objectives such as 'At the end of the course, participants will know about the physiology of respiration.' These are false objectives with a description of content with no specification about the learning outcomes. Therefore they do not fulfill the criteria of educational objectives.

Educational objectives are integral components of instructional planning and not to be seen in isolation. Good educational objectives have to be linked to instructional methods and assessment in order to improve the learning outcomes. In addition, we need to be aware of the relationship between higher order cognitive levels and much-desired problem solving skills. We should consciously and repeatedly practice to attain the skills necessary to formulate those 'higher order' educational objectives. Such educational objectives not only challenge the learners into critical thinking and problem solving but also force us to improve our teachings.

In summary, the important points that we have learned are

- Educational objectives are learner-centered, short, and precise descriptions of what learners are expected to achieve at the end of the program
- Good learning objectives include specifications about (a) target audience, (b) observable behavior, (c) condition, and (d) degree
- Educational objectives are directly linked to instructional methods and assessment and evaluation

References and Further Readings

1. Ramsden P. Learning to Teach in Higher Education. 1992. London: Routledge. Web address:
   http://www.usyd.edu.au/su/ctl/peter/Aims/object2.htm.
2. Schultheis NM. Writing Cognitive Educational Objectives and Multiple-Choice Test Questions. *American Journal of Health-System Pharmacists*. 1998; 55: 2397–401.

Section 6

Instructional
Methodologies: General

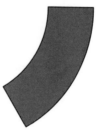
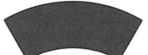
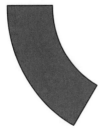

Assessment
and
evaluation

Educational
objectives

**Instructional
methodology**

10 Overview of Teaching and Learning Methods

I hear and I forget
I see and I remember
I do and I understand

Confucius, 551–479 BC

With this chapter, we begin to explore various teaching and learning methods that we can use to reach the learning objectives that we have discussed earlier. We emphasize incorporation of *learning* methods, alongside with more traditional teaching methods, in line with the spirit and philosophy that we want to promote.

Range of Teaching and Learning Methods

There are many teaching and learning methods to choose from. For our purpose we divide these methods into three categories: (a) expository, (b) exploratory, and (c) simulation. The *expository* method is the unidirectional delivery or presentation of information to the learner. The original verb is 'exposition', the literal meaning of which is to showcase. Traditional lecture, reading a book, or reading from the web generally involve passive transfer of information.

Exploratory methods prompt the learners to explore and discover by way of interactions. In contrast to expository method of learning, exploratory methods allow and encourage two-way exchange of information. Examples of exploratory forms of teaching and learning activities include discussion, question and answer, and brainstorming. Other adaptations of exploratory form are case-based and problem-based learning. *Simulation* is another category of teaching and learning method that allows practice of learned skills in safe situations that closely resemble real life. Simulation allows the careful and gradual transfer of learned skills into actual practice. Role-play and standardized patients are examples of simulation in medical education.

Type of Teaching and Learning Methods	Dominant Features	Illustrative Examples
Expository	Passive transfer of information	Lecture, reading a book
Exploratory	Discovery and exploration	Discussion, question and answer, case- and problem-based learning
Simulation	Practice of learned skill in safe environment	Role-play

Educational Effectiveness of Teaching and Learning Methods

The differences in educational effectiveness of these forms of teaching and learning are striking. Expository forms of teaching and learning methods, although generally more structured and allow orderly transfer of large amount of information, are significantly restricted in their abilities to bring meaningful change in educational experience. Information may be transferred efficiently but rarely remembered or utilized. Thus, expository methods must be supported with other forms of teaching and learning activities.

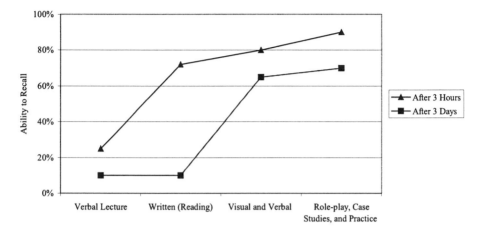

Fig. 1. Comparative effectiveness of teaching and learning methods. (Data from Dale, 1969)

The comparative effectiveness of these various forms of teaching is evident from several studies (Dale, 1969; Joyce and Shower, 1981). Lectures and other passive forms of teaching and learning methods are very inefficient in their ability to produce lasting impressions in the learner (Fig. 1). Without practice and opportunity for discussion, the information obtained is rapidly lost. Thus, learners typically recall only 25% of the information presented in a traditional lecture after three hours and about 10–20% after three days. In sharp contrast, participatory form of learning methods, such as role-play and case-studies, results in retention of 90% information after three hours and 70% information after three days (Dale, 1969).

The effectiveness of these various forms of teaching and learning methods in skill attainment and transfer of the skills to actual practice differs greatly as well. For example, only 10–20% of the skills that are taught in the form of theory are actually attained and an insignificant 5–10% of the skills are actually transferred into practice (Joyce and Shower, 1981). Encouragingly, with gradual incorporation of demonstration, practice, feedback, and coaching almost 80–90% of the skills can be attained and transferred into practice by the learners (Fig. 2).

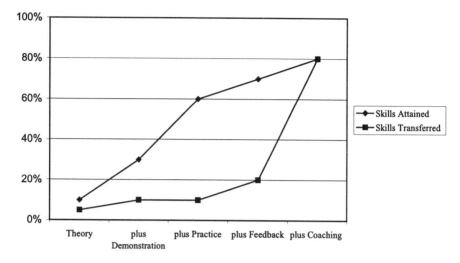

Fig. 2. Comparative effectiveness of teaching and learning methods in skill attainment and transfer (Data from Joyce & Showers, 1981)

This vividly illustrates the critical need to *transform passive forms of teaching to more active and interactive forms of learning.* The importance of active and interactive form of learning is fittingly described by the ancient Chinese proverb that is noted at the beginning of this chapter. We do not need to abandon more traditional form of teachings, such as lecture all together. We can promote desired active and interactive forms of learning even in the traditional teaching formats with simple but planned incorporation of various techniques.

Thus, we should *broaden our repository of teaching and learning methods.* Medical teachers, most of whom are taught in traditional paradigm and have very little exposure to many innovative teaching and learning methods, generally engage in few selected methods which almost universally include passive lecture. But medical education encompasses complex activities that are spread through all three domains of education: knowledge, attitude, and skills. The variation and complexity of learning objectives necessitate incorporation of a diverse range of learning methods. Teaching and learning methods vary in their ability for a particular task. There is no one single method that can meet the demands of all of our teaching and learning needs. Therefore, we should actively familiarize ourselves with many useful teaching and learning methods that medical education has to offer and judiciously use the most appropriate one for the learning objectives.

Organization of Chapters

The following chapters are organized as follows. The first few chapters discuss the more generic teaching and learning methods including lecture, small group, role-play, case-based teaching, questioning technique, and feedback. Subsequent chapters discuss clinical teaching including conceptual framework, effective delivery of clinical teaching, clinical reasoning, and teaching procedural and communication skills. Finally, there is a separate discussion on problem-based learning including PBL processes and implementation.

In summary, the key issues that we have learned are

- There are many teaching and learning methods which differ in their usefulness to achieve the demands of a particular task
- Traditional lecture and similar passive educational activities produce short-lived impact on the learners
- Transfer of learning into real-life improves progressively with active participation and practice

References and Further Readings

1. Dale E. Cone of Experience. In: *Education Media: Theory into Practice*. Wiman RV (Editor). 1969. Charles Merrill. Columbus, Ohio. USA.
2. Joyce B, and Showers B. The Transfer of Training: The Contribution of Coaching. *Journal of Education*. 1981. 163(2): 163–72.
3. McIntosh N. Why do We Lecture? JHPIEGO Strategy Paper. 1996. The Reproductive Online. The John Hopkins University. Web address: www.reproline.jhu.edu; accessed May 02.

11 Making Lecture Effective

If we are to be required to assess educational quality and learning by virtue of how long a student sits in a seat, we have focused on the wrong end of the student.

Laura Palmer Noone,
Testimony before Web-based Education Commission
Quoted in 'The Power of the Internet for Learning'

Lecture is the one of the most common forms of instruction in the medical schools. The ubiquitous presence of lectures is deeply ingrained in the academic culture. It is practiced in classrooms, seminars, in-hospital teaching, and in continuing medical education conferences. Recently, with growing popularity of learner-centered approaches in education, several questions have naturally surfaced regarding the appropriateness of lecture. Do lectures still have a role in medical education? What modifications are necessary that would make lectures more appropriate in the current model of learning and teaching?

In this chapter, our tasks are to

- Recognize the advantages and limitations of lectures
- Determine the situations where lectures are effective

- Create conceptual framework of lecture
- Propose changes in the traditional lecture format to make it more active and interactive

We make an argument that lecture can be effective and appropriate provided its *limitations are recognized and lectures are made to be more interactive*. We demonstrate how to transform the students from a state of *captive listeners* to *active contributors*.

Lecturing is one of the oldest forms of instruction. It is not merely a collection of information that the teacher delivers to the students. A series of well-constructed lectures represents an argument or a hypothesis. It is the teacher's effort to understand a large body of knowledge and synthesize and present the knowledge in a simplified manner to the students' level of understanding (Brinkley *et al*, 1999). Thus, the teacher's responsibility in a lecture also includes analysis, synthesis, selection of relevant information, and elimination of irrelevant ones. Properly done, the lecture is a creative and personal work by the teacher modeled upon his intellectual scaffolding. Few other forms of instructional method demand such a high degree of originality from the teachers, making it both challenging and rewarding for them.

Advantages

The most important advantage of lecture is the efficient and organized delivery of a large body of information. The lecture enables the teacher to deliver an impressive quantity of information to a relatively large number of students in a short period of time. These factors probably explain the high popularity of lecture as an instructional method. The utilization of materials and human resources is minimum compared to other instructional methods; making it especially attractive to administrators. Lectures also give a sense of control to the lecturers—an attribute that is often favored by many.

Advantages of Lecture

- Delivery of large body of content
- Addresses large audience group
- Minimum time and resource utilization
- Well structured and coherent
- Empowerment and sense of control by teachers

Limitations and Concerns

The greatest concern of lecture in its traditional form is that it puts the students in an *inactive and passive role*. Lectures, especially with large groups, seem to be at odds with prevalent learning theories and practice.

The behavior and role of the students and the teacher during a lecture appear to be modeled after our social expectations and hierarchy. Attending lecture is analogous to attending to a play. The audience's role is to enjoy the play and appreciate the actors and actresses. The audience is not expected to interrupt the play nor question the actors. A good play deserves applause when the actors play out their role properly. The style and showmanship often receive more attention than the content or the message. Similarly, the lecture can be viewed as a one-man-play with monologue by the teacher. If the teacher is a good performer, the students listen attentively but rarely interrupt to ask questions. The social expectations are not to raise issues that lead to discussion and clarification. The passivity of the students during lecture contradicts the practice of learner-centered learning approaches.

Passive form of lecture without students' participation is also very ineffective and usually fails to produce any lasting effects on the students. Very little information is remembered and most of it is lost after a short while. Higher levels of cognitive functions such as application, analysis and synthesis, are not practiced during lectures. Moreover, the lecture is not the most suitable method for teaching complex and advanced topics such as understanding of disease processes, decision making exercise, and elaborate diagnostics and therapeutic modalities.

Nevertheless, interactive and effective lecturing is possible with simple attention to planning and creativity.

Limitations of Lecture

- Lack of active participation
- Lack of long-term effects
- Limited suitability to cultivate higher order cognition
- Limited suitability for problem topics

Components

The fundamental organization of a lecture is similar to the familiar structure of a scientific paper. A basic lecture is organized in three main sections: (a) introduction, (b) body, and (c) conclusion.

Introduction

The first 5–10 minutes of the lecture is spent on introduction. Introduction is much more than outlining the contents of the topic. Introduction lays down the purpose, organization, and ground rules of the lecture. A useful way of organizing the introduction is to seek answers for the following questions:

- What are the most important features of the topic?
- What is the most important information that I want my students to know?
- What are the key concepts that I would like to share with the students?

- What are the questions that I would like to ask during this lecture?

Answers to these questions lay down the scaffolding upon which the rest of the lecture shapes up.

It is useful to prepare an introductory note to highlight the important points you have considered during this stage. For example, when preparing a lecture on diabetic ketoacidosis, you may want to emphasize the key teaching points by this remark: "Today we will discuss diabetic ketoacidosis—an acute complication of diabetes mellitus. Treatment of this life-threatening complication requires prompt identification of the clinical features and institution of treatment based on patho-physiology. So, in this lecture we will discuss the clinical features and the patho-physiological basis of management of this complication." Such introductory remarks help the students to concentrate on the important points of the lecture and grasp the core information efficiently.

The body

This is the major component of lecture when most of the information is presented. The body of the lecture contains, in addition to facts, arguments or concepts that have been presented during the introduction. The body may also contain illustrations with actual patients' story, pathological slides or X-rays to further such arguments. The content in the body progresses logically and coherently with clear sign-posting from one topic to another to bolster these arguments and concepts.

The first part of the body provides a broad overview of the topic—a simple concept for the learners to understand. Preferably, this formative section should not contain any controversial aspects or any premature qualifiers or conditions to the concept. The complicated and controversial topics, if necessary, are introduced later when the students are comfortable with the fundamentals. Alternative and competing viewpoints are important but should be introduced carefully without jeopardizing the basic concepts.

The conclusion

Every lecture contains a conclusion that includes a compelling and carefully selected take-home message for the students to remember. The take-home message is brief and succinct, yet powerful in content. A lengthy conclusion appears as another argument and erodes the key message. Alternatively, instead of straightaway providing them with the key messages, you may encourage the students to write down few important points that they have learned during the lecture and share those with the rest. The conclusion section should also direct the students to future readings and set aside specific time for question and answer.

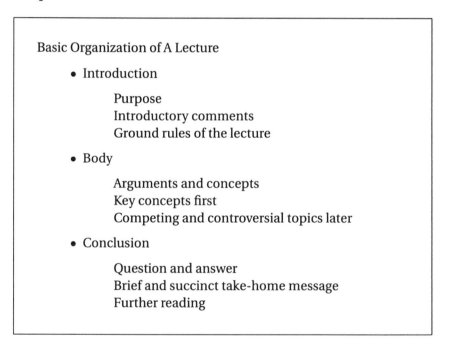

Basic Organization of A Lecture

- Introduction

    Purpose
    Introductory comments
    Ground rules of the lecture

- Body

    Arguments and concepts
    Key concepts first
    Competing and controversial topics later

- Conclusion

    Question and answer
    Brief and succinct take-home message
    Further reading

Ways to Make Lecture More Learner-Centered

As the major concern regarding lecture is the lack of audience participation; efforts are made to make lecture more participatory and interactive without making the structure and orderliness of lecture atmosphere vulnerable. There are simple innovations that can be adapted to individual lecture style.

Periodic pause and review

During the lecture, allow the learners with periodic short breaks every 10–15 minutes interval. During the pause, learners work in pairs to review, discuss, and revise their notes. Provision of such breathing space during the lecture allows the learners to assimilate, clarify, and strengthen their newly learned information (Bonwell and Eison, 1991).

Carefully crafted questions and answer

Judicious use of questioning during the lecture helps to promote active thinking. Questioning during lecture is done with specific purpose in mind. The idea is *not* to test the knowledge but to identify students' weakness, bring their attention to specific points, and generally encourage them into thinking. Questioning time does not have to be at the end of the lecture; it can be done during the lecture immediately before or after a key fact is presented as well. To maintain the organization and cohesiveness of the lecture, such questions need to be pre-planned and built around the theme of the lecture.

Immediate test

A simple test at the end of the lecture allows students to comprehend and retain learned information more quickly. Such tests are directly linked to the purpose of the lecture and highlight the important key points for the students to remember. The proximity of such tests after the lecture is important. Studies have shown that such immediate tests doubles the retention of information of the lecture materials compared to tests given several weeks later (Bonwell and Eison, 1991).

Study session

In this format, the main lecture is broken down into two more or less equal segments with an interval in between. During the interval students form small study groups and work around a study guide that contains several key questions. Students discuss the study questions and create new questions for answer. The study questions may include clinical problem solving exercises to determine the relevance and application of presented facts.

As we strive towards the learner-centered learning model, the role of and emphasis on lectures should continue to evolve. Traditional lectures with one-way passive delivery of information are almost sure to become extinct. The number of lectures should be reduced. The emphasis should be on making the remaining lectures more aligned with the learner-centered learning model by incorporating more interactive and stimulating exercise.

In summary, the important topics that we have learned are

- Lectures deliver a large amount of information to a sizeable number of audience
- A lecture is organized into basic sections of (a) introduction, (b) body, and (c) conclusion
- Lack of active participation from the students is the major limitation of traditional lecture
- Lectures can be made interactive and participatory without jeopardizing the structure and cohesiveness with simple innovations such as questioning and periodic pause and review

References and Further Readings

1. Bonwell CC, and Eison JA. Active Learning: Creating Excitement in the Classroom. *ERIC Digest.* 1991. ERIC_NO: ED340272.

ASHE-ERIC Higher Education Reports. The George Washington University, Washington, DC, USA.

2. Brinsky A, Dessants B, Flamm M, Fleming C, Forcey C, and Rothschild E. The Art and Craft of Lecturing. 51–64. In: *Chicago Handbook for Teachers: A Practical Guide to the College Classroom.* 1999. The University of Chicago Press. Chicago, IL, USA.

3. The Power of the Internet for Learning. Report of the Web-Based Education Commission to the President and the Congress of the United States. December 2000. Washington DC. USA.

12 Understanding Small Group

From the earlier discussion on teaching and learning concepts, we have recognized the importance of active nature of learning. We have also identified that learning is also a *social activity* that progresses through collaboration and interaction. Small group method is one of the ways to promote active and collaborative learning.

In this chapter, our tasks are to

- Identify the educational characteristics of small groups
- Discuss the advantages and implementation considerations
- Determine the role and responsibility of a small group leader

After completing the chapter, we will recognize the relevance and importance of small group as an instructional methodology and be able to function as an effective group leader.

Definition

A small group is a collection of several learners who *interact* and *work* together to achieve *common learning goals*. Interaction in small group is unrestrained and open and revolves around several norms and procedures. Such norms and procedures are reached either spontaneously or by consensus. Having common learning goals is critical for small group formation and is the major driving force for proper functioning of the group. Common learning goals bring structure and cohesiveness into the group and help in the development of collective responsibility among the group members.

The number of learners in the group varies. A minimum of three to four learners is necessary for the proper functioning of small groups. Two learners are inadequate to form a group and act more like a dyad. The presence of a large number of learners in a group is also detrimental to proper functioning of the group. Large numbers encourage formation of smaller sub-groups within the group. Most educators are probably comfortable with approximately five to ten students in each small group.

Advantages

The most important advantage of small groups is the ability of the small group to foster active and collaborative learning. These two characteristics are very important components in learner-centered learning approaches and supported by diverse theories such as constructivist theory, adult learning principles, and social learning theories. Active learning in the group is necessary to promote higher order cognitive processes such as analysis and problem solving.

The formation of a group fosters shared responsibility and teamwork and brings individual expertise into the group. Thus, a small group is able to execute more demanding and complicated work that would not have been possible by working in isolation. A small group creates an even playing field for the learners and eases the distinctions between the better learners and the less efficient ones.

Small groups have been used to support a wide range of learning activity. In line with the theoretical construct, small groups work best for those kinds of learning activity that require significant collaboration and collective exercise that is beyond the mastery of an individual learner. Examples of such demanding situations include project-based and case-based learning, dealing with complicated clinical scenarios, and complex diagnostic and decision making exercises. Small groups are used extensively in the problem-based curriculum.

Advantages of Small Groups

- Production of higher quality work
- Better decision-making than as individuals
- Undertake more complicated tasks or projects
- Integration of several learning processes such as talking, listening, writing, and reading
- Opportunity to experience and observe other group members
- Expand the repertoire of learning strategies
- Break down the isolation
- Ease the distinction between tutor and learners

Adapted with modifications from Susan Imel. Small Groups in Adult Literacy and Basic Education. 1992. EIRC Digest Number 130.

What is the advantage of using small group method over large group? The question is difficult to answer as the nature and quality of the group activity are more important factors that overshadow the issue of the number of learners in a group. Practice-based literature and anecdotes support small groups, but empirical evidence is scanty to support the notion that having small groups results in definite improvements in learning when compared to large groups. The general consensus is that small group does not have any overt advantage over large group to achieve knowledge acquisition but a properly functioning small group promotes active learning and in turn may make a difference in fostering higher order cognitive skills in the learners (Imel, 1992).

Challenges for Small Group

Proper functioning of small groups requires recognition of several important challenges and attributes of the group.

Variation of the learners

Group members differ from each other in their prior level of knowledge, educational interest, learning effectiveness, and ability to work within a group. While diversity promotes varied and interesting opinions, it also has the potential of creating conflicts and interfering with the proper functioning of the group.

Group leadership skills

Proper functioning of the group depends on a good group leader. Tutors vary in their ability to be a group leader which can be enhanced by proper training and practice.

Finding a common ground

Groups function properly when group members share common learning goals and have common expectations and roles. Difference in finding a common ground is an obstacle that groups have to overcome by negotiation.

Content and instructional materials

Learning activities in small groups are driven by the learners. Apart from text-books, a wide range of instructional materials are needed to satisfy diverse learning activities.

Time

The small group tutorial is a relatively slow process. The preparation time for small group activity is generally longer than that for other forms of tutoring.

Assessment

It is customary to assess each individual member of the group. Assessing the group's collective knowledge or skill in an objective manner has yet to find a place in the conventional curriculum.

Life Cycle of a Group

Small group formation and progression is a dynamic process and passes through several phases during its life. The following stages of life cycle are recognizable in a small group (Tubbs, 1995).

Orientation

This stage starts with the assignment of the problem. Group members familiarize with each other, identify their strengths and weaknesses. They start to formulate the learning goals and establish group etiquette and ground rules.

Conflict

This is the stage of creative tension and is essential for the group's productivity. Group members begin to test emerging hypotheses, critically analyze and evaluate each other's proposals.

Consensus

Consensus stage is reached when members compromise and bring an end to the conflict state. During the consensus stage group members judge alternative proposals and agree to a solution.

Closure

In this stage, the group consensus is further refined and crystallized in the form of a final result. The group members forego their differences and assert their support for the decision.

The life span of the group varies depending on several factors including complexity of the task. Although it is possible to complete a simple task in one session, several sessions are necessary for more complicated ones. The maturity of the group depends on the stability of the composition of the group members. If the composition of the group remains unchanged, the group tends to mature quickly and little time is spent in the orientation phase.

The phase of the group's life cycle has practical implications for the group leader. It is often prudent for the group leader to be more directive in leadership style during the initial stages of group formation. A more hands-off approach is better suited towards the final stages when the group's norm and procedures are well established.

Types of Group

The mere formation of small groups does not necessarily equate to proper functioning. The nature and scope of the task, clarity of the instructions, leadership skills, and group members' contributions are important factors in determining the functional ability of the group. The interplay of these factors leads to emergence of several recognizable categories of groups.

An ideal group is on-task where the group members are willing to share meaningful information and ideas with each other. Such groups maintain a sense of trust and function with a high level of expectations (Imel, 1992).

Less desirable groups are also formed during small group activity. Groups may remain on-task but fail to talk and listen and hinder exchange of meaningful ideas. A leaderless group fails to exchange ideas and does not progress towards the target. Sometimes, a completely dysfunctional group is formed with no participation from the group members.

An ideal group rarely forms spontaneously in the first place. There is a definite maturation process, self-reflection, and learning from the errors before a group becomes seasoned and productive.

Role and Responsibilities of Tutors in Small Groups

The role and responsibilities of the tutor in a small group assume two basic dimensions: (a) ensuring social cohesiveness in the group and (b) keeping the group on target. Both are important and connected with each other. Social cohesiveness and effective interactivity within the group ensure that the group remains on target and achieves the learning goals.

Role and Responsibility of Tutors in Small Group

- Determination of the purpose of the group
- Delegation of responsibility
- Help in maturation of small group
- Development of group norms and etiquette
- Resource identification
- Crisis resolution
- Promotion of reflection within the group
- Assessment of group's function

Small groups support a variety of teaching and learning activities in medical education. It is the predominant mode of learning in problem-based and project-based learning and complements other forms of learning activities as well. It is unlikely that small groups will completely replace lecture, one-to-one, and large group teaching. A more likely scenario is various forms of instructional methods will be in existence together, each addressing unique demands of the individual learning situation.

In summary, the key points that we have learned are

- Small group is formed when there are common learning goals
- Small group supports active and collaborative learning
- Variation in learning needs, style, and pace among the learners is a potential obstacle that needs to be overcome

- Group matures in identifiable phases: orientation, conflict, consensus, and closure
- An ideal group facilitates free exchange of ideas while remaining on target to fulfill the learning goals
- Tutors' responsibility in the group includes maintaining social organization and keeping the group on target

References and Further Readings

1. Borchers T. Moorhead State University. Small Group Communication. 1999. Web address: http://www.abacon.com/commstudies/groups/definition.html. Accessed in May 02.
2. Imel S. Small Groups in Adult Literacy and Basic Education. 1992. ERIC Digest No. 130. ERIC_NO: ED350490.
3. Tubbs S. A System Approach to Small Group Interaction. 1995. McGraw-Hill, New York, USA.
4. Westberg J and Jason H. Fostering Learning in the Small Groups: A Practical Guide. Springer Series on Medical Education. 1996. Springer Publishing Company. Broadway, NY, USA.

13 Case-Based Teaching

Case-based teaching is a common form of teaching and learning method in medical education. This form of teaching is effective in inculcating critical thinking, problem solving, and other higher order cognitive skills.

In this chapter, our tasks are to

- Discuss the educational rationale of case-based teaching
- Recognize the strengths and uses of case-based teaching
- Identify various types of case
- Determine the steps of selecting a suitable case
- Construct a sample teaching script for case-based teaching

The focus of this chapter is to provide an overview of case-based teaching. The case-based teaching in PBL and other specialized situations is discussed separately.

Definition

Simply speaking a case is a description of problem where the learners' task is to solve the problem. In medicine, case is often a description of patients' problem that requires analysis and interpretation of data and decision-making by the learners. The data of the problem may be submerged within the case or have to be gathered from other sources. Such sources of data can be very varied and may range from patients' story, physical examination findings, laboratory values, and even information obtained from published literature. The learners' tasks are to critically analyze the relevance and usefulness of the data, decipher their meaning, and eventually propose a hypothesis. The hypothesis proposition generally includes plan for an investigation, diagnosis of patient's problem, and suggestion for treatment.

Case-based teaching is one of the key instructional methods in medicine. Although, patient-bedside is the most familiar place for case-based teaching; with ingenuity and innovation case-based teaching can be practiced in other situations with the help of real or simulated paper-based cases. Paper-based cases are written case-scenarios that may or may not be derived from real cases.

Educational Rationale

The value of cased-based teaching lies in exploiting 'the basic human capacity to learn from stories' (Schank, 1994). Learning from stories is different from other forms of expository teaching such as lecture, reading, or demonstration where the data are well-constructed, unambiguous, and coherent in presentation. Learners do not have to struggle hard to interpret the data. In contrast, patient's story or case exposes the learners to unstructured situations characterized by ambiguity, absence of all information, and conflicting patients' problems. The challenges for the learners are to analyze and interpret the patient's problems and propose convincing solutions or explanations for these problems.

In medicine, information processing is a much-desired attribute of the learners. Learners are required to gather information, prioritize the information according to their importance and relevance, and filter-out irrelevant and redundant information. Eventually information processing directs towards solutions of the patient's problem or development of a management plan. In the process, learners also establish connections between the specifics of that particular case and experiences with other patients (Irby, 1994). This helps the learners to generalize the information learned from one particular case to other patients' problems.

Many of these functions require assumption of the role of decision-makers by the learners—a role often fought with apprehension and hesitancy. The feeling of apprehension is a major deterrent for free-thinking and full utilization of their cognitive processes. If the learners can be freed from the feeling of risk and tension, the learning would become more spontaneous, decisions and judgements would reflect their true thinking process. They are also more likely to venture beyond their comfort zones and experiment with challenging situations. Case-based teaching provides learners with simulated low-risk situations, a safe-haven, where they can assume the role of the clinicians and decision- makers.

Benefits of Case-Based Teaching

- Development of problem-solving skills
- Identification and prioritization of important information
- Identification of critical missing information
- Formulation of concise, reasonable and consistent patient management plans
- Presentation and defense of own ideas
- Influence and persuasion of others
- Examination of multiple points of views
- Creation of simulated situations
- Generalization of patient-specific data to other situations

---

Concerns for Case-Based Teaching

Concerns for case-based teaching include its potential unstructured nature of instruction and the lack of direction in the learning process. Learners and teachers alike may feel overwhelmed by the immensity of information and lose valuable time to sort out the details. Careful selection and planning of the case will mitigate some of these problems.

Variations of Cases for Teaching

Cases in medicine can assume varied dimensions depending on several factors. From the perspectives of teaching the most important of these factors are the goals of the session, and prior knowledge and level of understanding of the learners. Based on these factors, cases can be simple that are suitable for beginners to more complex descriptions of problem for advanced level learners.

Illustrative cases highlight fairly straightforward information with specific teaching points. Background cases convey information, provide factual data, and emphasize specific points within the case. More complex cases portray elaborate scenarios requiring extensive problem solving exercises. Other complex cases include such patient scenarios where main issues are submerged in a mass of data (i.e. history, physical examination findings, and laboratory investigations) and contain many external distracters. This type of cases engages the learners to select, organize, and interpret data in order to devise a decisive management plan.

Although, case-based teaching is generally conducted in one session, in selected situations and if time permits, the teaching can be spread to several sessions and critical information about the case may be revealed step-by-step to simulate real patient encounters.

Case-Selection

Careful selection of a case is an important first step that often determines the success of the session. Not every patient's scenario is useful for case-based teaching; nor do all the scenarios contain teaching points of interest. Several important decision points help in selecting suitable cases during teaching.

- *The level of understanding of the learners*: Ideal cases are neither too difficult nor too easy for the learners. For a group of learners who has just started clinical rotation a case with important historical or physical examination findings may suffice. For more experienced learners a case that demands complex diagnostic or decision making exercises is more appropriate.

- *Integration of concepts*: Integration of concepts from different disciplines or specialties allows learners to reinforce their learning and to develop broader perspectives about patient management. Often a case provides unique opportunity to integrate basic science, clinical science, and psychosocial aspects of medicine that are unattainable through textbooks. The possibility of integration of concepts should be explored in each case.

- *Open-ended*: Some patient scenarios are problem oriented with many unresolved and unsettled issues. This type of cases allows the learners to reach multiple interpretations and propose an assortment of solutions. Such cases also provide opportunities to advance discussions of several disease processes simultaneously.

The complexity and nature of the case vary with the need of the session and learners' prior educational background and knowledge. In the next page, we propose a scheme for choosing a case based on the level of the learners. The presented attributes may be viewed as a continuous spectrum, the teacher's responsibility is to choose the right 'color' that is best suited for the learner.

Preparing the Case for Teaching

Once the selection of the case is over, the case has to be prepared for teaching. The process is greatly simplified by answering the following questions:

Table 1. Selection of a case.

Beginner Level Learners	Advance Level Learners
Illustration of specific points	Comprehensive patient management
Well-structured	Ill-structured
Selected information	Redundant information
Focused on single aspect (medical or psychosocial)	Integration of psychosocial and ethical perspectives
Information is provided	Information is gathered

- What are the key issues of the case? What do I intend to achieve from the case? Does this case fit my teaching objectives?

  Every case has its own illustrative teaching points. It may be an important historical information, a unique physical examination finding, or a complex treatment plan that we want our learners to learn.

- What are the critical information of the case that are lacking? How can they be obtained (e.g. reviewing of old notes, contacting physicians)? Is the information complete enough to reach a reasonable conclusion by the learners?

  Often some pivotal information of the case is missing, making the whole process precarious and entirely hypothetical. Careful review of the patient case prior to the session alleviates the unwelcome surprise.

- What are the ideal solutions of the case? What are the feasible alternatives?

  Rarely a clinical case will 'read the text book' and present in a typical fashion. This is an opportunity to explore the ideal as well as alternative and competing solutions (diagnosis, plan of investigations, and therapy) of the case.

- What information should be available to the students at the beginning? What should be available to them in the later part of discussion?

  Some key information will help the learners to focus on the case. Unless there are some specific pedagogical reasons such

key information should be provided early in the session.
- What are the questions I am going to ask? When am I going to use these questions?

  The success of case-based teaching depends on carefully crafted questions that should be thought of during the development of the case. Questioning can direct the discussion and can keep the group on track towards solving the problem. Conversely, poor quality questions may tempt the students just to answer the questions deviating from their role as decision-makers.

Based on the above questions and answers, we should be able to create a script for case-based teaching. The script contains the essential information about the case that directs the learning in the session. Creation of such scripts brings organization and structure into the session that greatly improves the success of the case-based teaching.

Script for Case-Based Teaching
Minimum Information

Content area

Key learning issues

Opening statements explaining
- Reasons for choosing the case
- Ground rules
- Expectations from the learner

Key questions that are to be asked

A concluding remark reiterating
- What has been learned
- How the information can be applied to other situations

Case-based teaching is a distinctive form of teaching and learning experience. Each case is unique and is capable of providing valuable learning opportunities. Careful planning and preparation improve the chance of success in case-based teaching.

In summary, the important points that we have learned are

- Case-based teaching inculcates critical thinking and problem solving abilities
- Selection of a case is based upon the goal of the session and learners' prior level of understanding
- Ill-structured cases are more suitable for advanced learners whereas beginners benefit more from simple illustrative cases
- Script for case-based teaching provides direction of learning and brings in structure to the session

References and Further Readings

1. Irby DM. What Clinical Teachers in Medicine Need to Know. *Academic Medicine*. 1994. 69 (5): 333-42.
2. Irby DM. Three Exemplary Models of Case Based Teaching. *Academic Medicine*. 1994. 69 (12): 947-53.
3. Schank RC. Active Learning through Multimedia. 1994. Spring. IEEE Multimedia, 69–77.

14 Role-Play

Education of the physicians is not limited to teaching and learning about medical knowledge; it also involves development of correct attitudes, behavior, and interpersonal and communication skills. Conventional teaching and learning methods, including lectures, are severely handicapped in teaching and learning of these essential attributes. Role-play is the preferred instructional method to instill attitudes and behavior and to develop the aforementioned skills.

In this chapter, our tasks are to

- Recognize the educational principles and rationale of role-play
- Discuss the correct usage and implementation process of role-play
- Critically review and analyze examples of role-playing scripts

After completing the chapter, we will be able to include role-play in our repository of instructional methods and conduct role-play session in an effective manner.

Role-play is a relatively unorthodox yet powerful teaching and learning activity where the learners act according to a simulated scenario. Typically, it involves two students; one of them acts as a patient and the other acts as a physician. Their play is based on defined learning objectives and well-crafted scripts. The audiences actively observe the role-play with predetermined criteria.

Advantages

The educational rationale of role-play capitalizes on several well-acknowledged principles. Role-play *actively engages* the learners in their learning activities. The learners not only learn about the topic, but actually get an opportunity to practice what has been learned. The learners are able to practice in a *safe environment* without fear of exposing their weaknesses and vulnerabilities. Thus, they are more likely to experiment and practice diverse skills beyond their usual comfort zones.

Role-play also *empowers* the learners to take control of the learning situations. It encourages generation of self-suggestions and helps in behavior modification. The material resource utilization during role-play is less as compared to other instructional methods.

Role-play brings *reality* to the teaching and learning. Learning is more effective if it takes place in an environment that closely resembles what are being taught. For example, the preferred way of teaching counseling techniques or interviewing skill is creating a situation where learners can actually *practice* these skills. The likeness with the actual situation also makes the transfer of skills to real-life much easier. Role-play is one of the ways of creating reality in a safe manner.

Advantages of Role-play

- Active participation of the learners
- Practice of learned skills
- Practice in safe environment
- Generation of self-suggestions

- Modification of behavior
- Taste of real-life scenarios
- Limited resource utilization

Applications

The major use of role-play in medical education is teaching and learning of communication and counseling techniques. It is also useful in situations where a desired behavior and attitude needs to be modeled or an existing behavior needs to be changed. With ingenuity, role-play can be utilized for peer-teaching and teaching psychomotor skills.

Example of counseling focused role-play session includes teaching medical students how to counsel diabetic patients regarding diet, medication usage, and recognizing hypoglycemia. Examples of psychomotor skill teaching where role-play is effective include demonstration of physical examination. In such scenarios, a pair of students plays the role of a teacher and a student and may use an anatomic model to demonstrate to each other the correct examination techniques. Scripts for these two specific scenarios are presented at the end of this chapter.

Examples of Usage of Role Play

- Interview technique
- History taking
- Counseling
- Negotiation of treatment
- Breaking bad news
- Peer teaching

Implementation Considerations

There are several important factors to be considered before choosing role-play as an instructional method. The common uneasiness is that role-play is a potentially unstructured activity. There are elements of disorganization that threaten the learning environ and can create chaos. Teachers are particularly uneasy about the potential disorganization as they believe this would lead to loss of control over the situation.

Many medical teachers voice concern about using this method for fear of inadequate coverage of content and insufficient training of the teachers. These are genuine concerns but fortunately they are surmountable with careful planning and preparation.

Learners' non-participation during role-play is another common concern. Quite expectedly, not every student feels comfortable in performing a role in front of an audience. But with encouragement and repeated role-play, the initial inhibition can be overcome and learners' participation gradually improves.

The Process

The success of role-play depends on careful planning and implementation. The planning phase is especially important to bring a desired level of structure and to make the process educationally meaningful.

In a role-play there are two or more actors, several observers, and a teacher. Actors role-play out according to scripts. In the process, they also learn from each other and provide feedback to the other. Observers actively watch the play usually with the help of predetermined criteria and provide feedback to the role-player. The teacher's responsibilities are to prepare the role-playing scripts, keep the play in focus, and active observation. The teacher is also responsible for targeted discussion at the end that includes a summary of the session, emphasis on what has been learned, how the process can be applied to real-life situations, and what could have been done better.

The script of the role-play is organized into the following sections:

• *Content coverage and goals of the session*

The script for the role-play should start by describing the content area that is to be covered during the role-play as well as clearly defined objectives.

• *Problem definition*

This segment lays down the scenarios of the role-play for all the players. This should include background problems, presenting problems, and potential sources of conflicts.

• *Instructions to role-players*

This section details the ground rules for the role-players including how the roles should be played, what should be the emphasis of the session, suggested time frame, and any other special instructions.

• *Instructions to the audience*

Similarly, this section describes the audiences' role during and after the role-play and the usage of check-lists (if any).

Tips on successful role-play

- Choose a case that simulates real-life scenarios that students are likely to encounter
- Inform learners beforehand that they are expected to role-play
- Inform learners what they are expected to learn from the role-play (objectives)
- Allow at least 3-5 minutes for players to read the scripts and prepare for the role

- Keep the instructions as specific as possible
- Instruct learners not to veer away from the focus of role-play
- Unless there is a specific pedagogical reason, ask role-players to sit
- Instruct learners to stay in their respective roles until the role-play is over
- Limit role-play to five to ten minutes. It can be exhausting!

Example of Scripts for Role-play: Counseling Focused

Content Area: Adult diabetic counseling at discharge
Goals: At the end of the role-play the learner will be able to

(a) Create a contingency plan for the patient in case of hypo-glycemia
(b) Demonstrate proper and safe use of anti-diabetic medications

Problem definition

Clinician's role: Dr. Adrian Tan is a family practitioner in Toa Payoh. He knows the patient Ms Ang.
Patient: Ms Ang is a 46 year old widow who lives alone. Both of her children are overseas pursuing their studies. She works as an office secretary. She has been diagnosed with mild diabetes for the last five years and is controlling her diet as per her doctor's advice. She has never taken any anti-diabetic medications. Recently she had a bout of pneumonia and was admitted to the Tan Tock Seng Hospital. The doctors in TTSH suggested that she should start taking oral-hypoglycemic medications. She learned from the Internet that such medications have many side effects. Her greatest fear is low

blood sugar and the possibility of 'passing out'. She is afraid that nobody will recognize this problem and she may die from that.

Focus of the role-play (to be read out to the role-players and audience)

The focus of this role-play is on the counseling technique of the doctor. The doctor needs to assess patient's understanding of the disease process and knowledge and possible misconceptions about oral hypoglycemic agents. The doctor needs to explore the extent of the social support system that the patient has. The doctor needs to discuss the signs and symptoms of hypoglycemia and suggest a plan detailing what should be done in case of hypoglycemia.

Role of observers

Please carefully observe role-players and focus on following questions.

(1) How did Dr. Tan approach Ms Ang? How effectively did he use questioning techniques to obtain Ms Ang's history?
(2) How effective was Dr Tan in explaining signs and symptoms of hypoglycemia? Did he consistently use terms that are understandable by a layman? Did he stop sufficiently and ask about Ms Ang's understanding? Did he propose a reasonable plan?

Example of Scripts for Role-play: Clinical Skill Practice

Content Area: Female pelvic examination
Goals: At the end of role-play, the students will be able to

(a) Examine the female pelvis according to the prescribed procedure in a manikin
(b) Identify the common anatomical landmarks in female pelvis

Scenario:

First student: You assume the role of a clinical supervisor for the fourth year medical students. Today's topic is examination of female pelvis. You recognize this is a sensitive issue. You are sufficiently conversant with the anatomy and were taught about the examination procedure by your clinical tutors. Your role today is to be a clinical teacher and you will teach students the correct procedures of female pelvic examination.

Second student: You will assume the role of a student and follow the instructions of the tutor. You will also practice yourself the examination process and return the demonstration to your tutor.

Note: Role reversal is an additional teaching technique where students will take turns to be a tutor and students. You may ask the students to conduct the examination just like they are expected to do in real life: introduce themselves, explain the procedure and findings to the patient, and maintain patient's privacy and confidentiality.

Role of the observers:

Please observe the role-play and focus on the following issues.

(1) Did the tutor introduce himself and the student to the 'patient'? Did he explain the procedures to the 'patient'?

(2) Did the tutor adequately explain and demonstrate the examination process to the students? Were the steps accurate?

In summary, the key concepts that we have learned in this chapter are

- Role-play actively engages the learners and empowers them to take control of their own learning
- Role-play is especially effective in learning counseling and communication skills
- Lack of structure and direction in learning are major barriers that needs to be addressed during role-play

- A script for role-play includes description of content coverage, purpose, problem definition, instructions to role-players and observers
- Teachers' responsibilities in role-play include keeping the play in order, active observation, and feedback

References and Further Readings

1. Bonwell CC, and Eison JA. Active Learning: Creating Excitement in the Classroom. *ERIC Digest.* 1991 ASHE-ERIC Higher Education Reports. The George Washington University. Washington, DC 20036-1183. USA. ERIC_NO: ED340272.
2. Reproductive Online. John Hopkins University. Baltimore. MD. Web address: http://www.reproline.jhu.edu/english/5tools/5tools.htm; accessed May 02.

15 Questions and Questioning Technique

To question well is to teach well. In the skillful use of questions, more than anything else, lies the fine art of teaching.

Earnst Sachs

Good questioning is an excellent aid to teaching that is seldom utilized to the fullest extent. Most of us use questioning solely to assess students' knowledge and are less aware of its expanded value as an important teaching and learning tool. Good questioning is a major determinant of teaching and learning outcomes.

In this chapter, our tasks are to:

- Recognize the importance of good questioning
- Discuss various types of questions with examples
- Determine the necessity of wait-time during questioning

After completing the chapter, we should be able to diversify our questioning techniques and seize the many unexplored advantages of good questioning.

Teaching scenario: You are about to precept final-year medical students in a pediatric inpatient ward. You have chosen Anna for case-based discussion. Anna is a four-month old Down syndrome patient with presenting symptoms of respiratory distress. You have already decided the principal goal of the session: students should be able to generate the differential diagnosis of respiratory distress in a four-month old child and differentiate between these conditions.

A question refers to any sentence, regardless of grammatical form, intended to elicit an answer (Caesin, 1995). Consider these two examples: 'What is the commonest chromosomal abnormality in Down syndrome?' and 'List the common causes of respiratory distress in the newborn.' Regardless of the difference in grammatical construction both sentences share a common intention of generating a response from the students—i.e. an answer—and therefore qualify as questions. Thus, an answer is defined as any response that fulfills the expectation of the question (Caesin, 1995). Closed-ended questions require selection from a limited range of choices, whereas, open-ended questions allow students more latitude to choose answers.

The purpose of questioning in medical education is manifold. Good questions during teaching (a) help students to participate actively in lessons, (b) provide an opportunity to students to express their ideas and thoughts, and (c) allow students to hear divergent opinions from fellow students. They draw attention to and highlight important points in the teaching and develop confidence and feeling of success in the students leading them beyond the conventional patterns of thinking. Good questions also help teachers evaluate their students' learning and thus revise the lessons as necessary.

Despite the fact that good questioning effectively improves learning, studies show that proper questioning is seldom practiced in teaching. Two main reasons for this lack are based on mistaken assumptions that questioning distracts the students from the lessons and creates undue anxiety for both students and teachers. On the contrary, proper questioning techniques help teachers to remain focused and create a conducive learning environment.

On the positive side, however, physicians are generally well-versed in questioning techniques. We use questioning every day with our patients that often starts with a few open-ended questions to elicit a range of responses. Questions like "How have you been in the last couple of months?" or "What can I do for you today?" are used to open the interview. Progressively, the questioning becomes more probing to seek clarification, broadening, or justification of prior issues and may involve selective use of close-ended questions. This pattern of progression and selection of different types of questions are analogous to many questioning techniques during teaching.

Types of Question

From educational viewpoint, several different types of questions are recognizable based on the intentions of the questions and nature of the anticipated answers.

1. *Factual questions* are used to get information from the students and often test rote memory.

Example: "What is the commonest chromosomal abnormality in Down syndrome?"

2. *Clarification questions* intend to provide clarity to both students and teachers. Such questions have important clueing effects and help students to revisit their earlier statements with alternative perspectives. We may use any of these as clarifying questions: "What do you mean by ..?" "Can you give me an example?" "Can you rephrase what you have just said?"

Example: "You mentioned possible thyroid problem contributing to Anna's symptoms. What do you mean by 'thyroid problem'? Can you give us an example?"

3. *Broadening or extension questions* enlarge the existing theme, explore implications of the response and can be useful in opening up further possibilities. Such questions can be used to assess additional knowledge of the students.

Example: "Do you know of any other chromosomal abnormality in Down syndrome?"

4. *Justifying questions* probe for assumptions and explore reasons for particular answers. These questions require significant comprehension and reasoning skills on the part of the students.

Example: "You mentioned respiratory tract infection as the most likely cause of Anna's breathing difficulty. What are your reasons for such a diagnosis?"

5. *Hypothetical questions* are used to explore students' understanding of complex situations beyond the scope of a particular encounter by creating hypothetical scenarios. Hypothetical questions often come in handy during the later part of teacher-student interactions when the basic facts and concepts are already established.

Example: "Suppose Anna has a ventricular septum defect and is taking diuretics to control her symptoms, how would you revise and rearrange the differential diagnosis of Anna's respiratory distress?"

6. *Questions about questions* probe for reasons for the question that students ask patients or teachers. This allows the students to verbalize their reasoning and understanding of the events leading to their own questions.

Example: "You asked Anna's mother whether Anna is taking any thyroid medications. Why did you ask that particular question? What are you thinking of?"

7. *Redirected questions* address the same question to several students and distribute responsibility. The benefits of such questions include generation of a wider variety of responses and allowing the students to evaluate each others' contributions. This technique shifts the focus from teacher-student interactions to *student-student interactions*.

Note that several of these question types, especially justifying questions, hypothetical questions, and questions about questions, encourage the students to engage in critical thinking and utilize educational objectives with higher cognitive values.

As we recognize the various question types and reflect upon our own teaching we may be able to identify that many of our questions during teaching are in fact 'list questions' that require recall of previously memorized information. We seldom utilize the full range of question types. Unfortunately, list questions are relatively easy to formulate and curricula sadly over-emphasize factual information over critical thinking. Such low cognitive level questions limit students' learning by not helping them to acquire a deep, elaborate understanding of the subject matter. List questions often start with 'when', 'where', 'who' and similar words that generate a closed response. In contrast, higher order questions require synthesis of information, force the students to reflect critically on the topic, develop reasoning skills and thereby, instill much deeper understanding of the topic. One simple way of avoiding questions that will lead to mere repetition of facts is the careful selection of words and verbs including some selected verbs from Bloom's classifications (Table 1). Examples of such words include: why, how, justify (as in 'justify your statements'), describe, defend, elaborate etc. Let us compare and contrast these examples:

- "What is the commonest cardiac abnormality in Down syndrome?"
- "Suppose Anna has the cardiac problem that you just mentioned, can you discuss the anticipatory advice that you would provide Anna's mother?"

Both questions are important, but the second question requires students to think deeply beyond recall of simple facts and is pedagogically sounder.

Dealing with Students' Wrong Responses

It is to be expected that during question and answer sessions, students will answer incorrectly, make wrong assumptions, and may

Table 1. During questioning

Use less of	Use more of
What	Why
When	How
Where	Suppose
Who	Justify
Which	Defend
	Elaborate

not be able to answer the question at all. Frequently students fail to answer the question not because they do not know the answer but because the question itself may be unclear to them. In such cases, rephrasing and simplifying the question is all that is needed to elicit correct answer.

When students fail to answer any question, ask them the following:

- Is the question clear to you?
- Do you want me to rephrase the question?
- Which part of the question did you not understand?
- Is the question too difficult for you?

Teachers are responsible for correcting mistakes and guiding the students in the proper direction. These are delicate moments in teacher-student interactions and deserve to be dealt with carefully. The teacher's dilemmas in these situations vary from inclination to favor discovery learning in the form of continuing guided questioning to adopting a more humane stance by maintaining silence or responding in a neutral manner. With careful probing and guiding questions it may be possible to elicit the correct response, but there are risks of potential embarrassment and eventual damage to the teacher-student relationship. Adopting a more humane approach, although more compassionate and sympathetic, is unlikely to correct the students' wrong responses and is pedagogically inadequate. Ende *et al* explored teachers' strategies of correcting wrong answers during clinical encounters and identified four possible strategies to deal with incorrect responses (Ende *et al*, 1995):

- Providing 'opportunity space' for revisions by not responding immediately and thus allowing the student time to come up with another answer
- Asking subsequent questions in a manner that contain clues to the first question leading the student to the correct answer
- Re-framing the questions so that the wrong answers become correct, and
- Treating the wrong answer as plausible but in need of further elaboration and consideration

These are useful approaches for the teachers to deal with situations when the students answer wrongly. Careful utilization of these approaches improves the chance of getting a correct answer from the students without jeopardizing the treasured harmony of teacher-student interactions.

Use of Silence

Some call it laziness. I call it deep thought.

Garfield©

Good questioning skills should also incorporate *proper use of silence*. As busy teachers we tend to interrupt the students right after a question is asked. The interruption may come in many forms: providing answers for the question, asking another question, providing own opinion, or even worse, outright criticism of the students' silence. It is rather illuminating to know that during typical teacher-student encounters, teachers rarely wait for more than 1.5 seconds after asking a question before interfering! (Tobin, 1987). As we promote and practice higher order cognitive questioning the use of silence becomes even more crucial. Unlike rote memory based questions, these higher order questions require significant mental processing by the students before any meaningful answer can be provided. So the period of apparent inactivity or 'wait time' is much needed.

Studies have documented that if the students are provided with even a modest increase of wait time, the length and correctness of their responses improve. They tend to be more forthcoming in providing answers, and the number of 'no answers' diminishes. Students are also more likely to produce high quality answers that commensurate with their higher cognitive abilities (Tobin, 1987).

Wait time benefits the teachers as well. With wait time, questioning strategies tend to be more varied and flexible and the number of questions decreases in quantity and increases in quality.

While we have discussed the benefits of wait time after the question is asked, a period of silence is also valuable after the students have *answered* the question. A brief period of silence at this point allows the students to reflect on what they have just said and permits us to consider their points thoroughly. It also conveys the important and much-needed message to the students about our attentiveness to their contributions.

The Benefits of Silence
For the students

- More meaningful answers
- Improved accuracy
- Improved length
- Fewer 'no answers'

For the teachers

- Higher order questions
- Precise formulation of questions
- Varied and flexible questions
- Convey teachers' attentiveness

Conscious effort is needed on our part to make use of silence as a part of routine questioning strategies. Although there is no prescribed length for the wait time, depending upon the complexity of the question and the students' expected level of understanding, 10 to 15 seconds of silence seems to be adequate. This time corresponds roughly to three complete breaths or slowly counting from one to ten or fifteen.

Question Cycle

Ask the question
↓
Period of silence
↓
(No response
↓
Simplify the question)
↓
Students answer
↓
Period of silence
↓
Discuss the answer

Needless to say, bad questioning is detrimental to learning. The effectiveness of a question is determined by both the content and the way the question is asked. Thus, questions that commensurate with students' level of understanding, are high in clarity, and when accompanied by a period of silence, are likely to be successful. As we consciously practice these simple questioning techniques we will be able to create a learning environment where higher order thinking is expected and practiced.

In summary, we have learned that

- Good questioning is a major determinant of the success of teaching

- Justifying questions, clarification questions, hypothetical questions, and questions about the questions are better in promoting higher order thinking skill
- Failure of the student to respond to a particular question is often due to the lack of his understanding of the question
- A period of silence after a question is asked and after a response is given is essential

---

Tips on Effective Questioning During Teaching

- Phrase questions clearly and succinctly
- Ask questions with specific intention
- Allow ten to fifteen seconds of wait time after asking a question before requesting a student's response
- Encourage students to respond even if they are wrong
- Probe students' responses to help them clarify ideas, reasoning process, or expand on their thinking
- Do not make automatic assumption that failure to answer the question is due to ignorance
- Acknowledge correct responses from students
- Make conscious efforts to ask higher cognitive order questions

---

References and Further Readings

1. Casein WE. Answering and Asking Questions. IDEA Paper No. 31. Manhattan, KS: Center for Faculty Evaluation and Development in Higher Education. *ERIC Online.* 1995.
2. Ende J, Pomerantz A, and Erickson F. Preceptors' Strategies for Correcting Residents in an Ambulatory Care Medicine Setting: A Qualitative Analysis. *Academic Medicine.* 1995; 70 (3): 224–9.
3. Sachs E. Quoted in: *Medical Education: A Surgical Perspective.* Edited by Bartlett RH. 1986. Lewis Publishers Inc. MI. USA.

4. Tobin K. The Role of Wait Time in Higher Cognitive Level Learning. *Review of Educational Research*. ERIC Clearinghouse on Reading and Communication Skills. 1987; 57 (1): 69–95.

16 Providing Effective Feedback

During teaching and learning activities information is obtained about performance, strengths, and weaknesses of the students. This information needs to be *transmitted* to the students in a manner that will bring the intended changes in their behavior. Feedback allows the transmission of information in an effective way.

In this chapter, our tasks are to

- Discuss the importance of feedback as an educational process
- Differentiate between praise and feedback
- Highlight the characteristics of good feedback
- Demonstrate with examples how these characteristics can be applied to teaching
- Discuss feedback in group situations

Feedback is a communication technique in which the teacher provides information to the students about their progress in mastering certain skills or achieving learning objectives of the course. In the setting of clinical education, feedback refers to information describing students' or house officers' performance in a given activity that is intended to guide their future performance in that same or in a related activity (Ende, 1983).

Despite the well-known association between effective feedback and improvement in learning, studies have shown it is seldom practiced. Moreover, often feedback is provided, unwillingly, in an ineffective and inappropriate manner. The paucity of feedback and its improper delivery are detrimental to teaching and learning. It leaves undesirable behavior uncorrected and even worse, may reinforce wrong and unacceptable behavior.

The reasons that are cited for the reluctance on providing feedback are many. One often quoted argument is that feedback potentially damages the rapport between the students and teachers, especially if such feedback involves negative ones. On the contrary, feedback that is provided with the intention of improving learning and in an appropriate manner is rarely misinterpreted by the student and actually strengthens the teacher-student relationship.

Educational Rationale

Feedback is an essential component of teaching and learning that connects instruction and assessment. During teaching and learning activities, students are continually assessed on their performance and the teacher's observation and interpretation of their performances have to be conveyed back to them systematically. The process ensures that they know what is right about them and what needs to be improved. Thus, feedback is about reinforcing and reiterating commendable behavior as well as correcting and improving the wrong ones.

Distinguishing Feedback from Praise and Criticism

Praise and criticism are not equivalent to feedback. From an educational viewpoint there are distinct and important differences. Praise and criticism are more like general comments about the person. They lack the description of specific behavior and its salutary or detrimental effects on the student.

Let us consider this example. You have noticed your student has gently escorted an elderly lady to the clinic during clinical encounter. A comment like "You did a good job" is more like praise. A proper feedback, on the other hand, would go beyond this simple praise and describe the specific behavior, its effects, and how it can be utilized in future. With this understanding it is easy to rephrase the praise and reconstruct it to a proper feedback. Following message is more likely to be effective and constitutes an example of proper feedback: "I noticed that you have volunteered to escort the lady to the room. This will definitely put the lady at ease. Remember this is exactly the kind of behavior that builds the essential rapport between the doctor and the patients." Note 'volunteer to escort' is the description of the behavior and the outcome of the behavior is 'put the lady at ease'. The next sentence with '... builds the essential rapport between the doctor and the patients' demonstrates to the students how they can utilize the specific commendable behavior in future.

Three Essential Elements in a Feedback Statement
Good Behavior

1. Description of the behavior
2. The salutary effects it has
3. How this can be utilized in future

Bad Behavior

1. Description of the behavior
2. The negative effects it has
3. How this can be avoided in future

Nature of Good Feedback

If we remember that the aim of the feedback is to improve and help students' learning, it is possible to agree on some general guidelines on the nature of good feedback (Stewart, 1995; Ende,1993; Kaprielian and Gradison, 1998).

- Good feedback tends to be *descriptive* rather than evaluative. It describes what is being observed. It is not aimed at entailing any judgement as to the performance or knowledge of the student.

  Example of descriptive feedback: You have obtained a good history of this patient with chest pain; but I noticed that you did not explore the cardio-vascular risk factors such as smoking, dietary habits or lifestyle.

  Avoid: You are rather weak in your interview skills.

- Good feedback is also *specific* rather than general. A good feedback points to the specific behavior or action on the part of the student. When the students recognize such specific behavior, they are more likely to incorporate that behavior. Conversely, a vague ambiguous statement sends mixed messages and creates confusion in the student.

  Example of specific feedback: You did rather well in obtaining details about family support but came short of asking the patient about his expectations on home management.

  Avoid: You have to improve on your patient management skills.

- An effective feedback technique addresses the *behavior or action* rather than the trait or character of the student. The students are more likely to be receptive if they understand that they are not the target of the feedback.

  Example of behavior or action focused feedback: I have observed that you did not introduce yourself or greet the patient. These prevented her from telling you much important information about her depression.

  Avoid: You were not interested in your patient.

- Feedback involves two-way *information exchange* between the teacher and the student. It is more of a dialogue where information is shared and common grounds are agreed upon. Thus, the teacher should frequently prompt the students who are encouraged to express their own views.

  Examples of prompter: What do you think about the interview that has just finished? Would you like to elaborate how the interview technique can be further improved?

- Good feedback ensures that students *understand the purpose* of the feedback. Thus, the teacher should frequently clarify the nature and objective of the feedback and actively solicit students' view about their understanding of the issues involved.

    Examples: Do you understand why I have given you the feedback? Is there anything that I can make clearer?

It is useful to set-aside *specific time* for feedback during a teaching session. This allows the teacher and the student to prepare adequately for the feedback and ensures feedback is conducted in a structured manner and with due seriousness. If possible, the time should be *soon after the encounter* between teacher and student so that a more detailed analysis of the events is possible when it is still fresh in memory.

A good habit is to *write down in exact verbatim* the key phrases and issues of the feedback and practice these beforehand. This is particularly helpful during difficult situations when unintended and careless words would make significant negative impact on students' learning.

Guidelines for Giving Feedback

- Feedback should be undertaken with the teacher and trainee working as allies with common ground
- Feedback should be well-timed and expected
- Feedback should be based on first-hand data
- Feedback should be regulated in quantity
- Feedback should be limited to those aspects of behavior that are remediable
- Feedback should offer subjective data and be labeled as such
- Feedback should deal with decisions and actions, rather than assumed intentions and interpretations

Adopted with minor modifications from Ende J. Feedback in Clinical Medical Education. *Journal of American Medical Association*. 1983. 250 (6): 777–81. Copyright © (1983), American Medical Association. All rights reserved. Used with permission.

Feedback in Group Settings

Feedback in a group situation can be precarious, as there is a risk of exposing individual student's vulnerability to others. This can be alleviated by careful incorporation of self-assessment and self-suggestion first and then progressively probe for the deficiencies.

The recommended sequence involves the following steps:

(1) Ask the student what she thinks she did right
(2) Ask the remaining students in the group what they think the student did right
(3) Ask the student what she did not do right. Ask how she can correct herself
(4) Finally ask the remaining students in the group what they think the student did not do correctly and solicit their opinion how the student could have done better

Following this sequence in exact order allows the students to explain their own strengths and provides opportunity of self-correction without exposing them to harsher criticism. This creates an ambience of greater receptivity and reduces embarrassment of the students.

Regular practice of all these specific attributes and recommendations is possible and practical. Good feedback comes naturally during teaching encounter with better understanding of the educational rationale of feedback and conscious incorporation of the aforementioned characteristics.

In summary, the important concepts that we have learned are

- Feedback is an educationally sound way of communicating teachers' observations to the students
- Feedback differs from criticism and praise and is more specific and descriptive
- The focus of feedback is behavior change and not judgement
- Feedback in group situations should include soliciting self-assessment and self-suggestion first

References and Further Readings

1. Ende J. Feedback in Clinical Medical Education. *Journal of American Medical Association*. 1983. 250(6): 777–81.
2. Kaprielian VS, and Gradison M. Effective Use of Feedback. *Family Medicine*. 1998. 30 (6): 406–7.
3. Stewart M, Brown JB, Weston WW, McWhinney IR, McWilliam CL, and Freeman TR. *Patient Centered Medicine: Transforming the Clinical Method*. 1995. Sage Publication. Thousands Oaks, California, USA.

Section 7

Instructional Methodology: Clinical Teaching

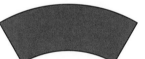

Assessment
and
evaluation

Educational
objectives

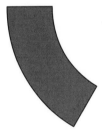
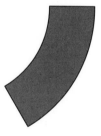

**Instructional
methodology**

17 Conceptual Framework for Clinical Teaching

Clinical teaching is the mainstay of teaching and learning in medicine. Close to 50% of teaching and learning activities during the undergraduate clinical years take place in the context of clinical teaching.

In this chapter, our tasks are to

- Identify the educational characteristics of clinical teaching
- Discuss precepting model in the context of clinical teaching
- Demonstrate a framework for needs identification and targeted teaching
- Define the attributes of an effective clinical teacher

Educational Characteristics of Clinical Teaching

How does clinical teaching differ from other forms of teaching? What are the special attributes of clinical teaching that are educationally important? The general principles of teaching and learning are applicable in clinical teaching as well; but there are a few important differences that have significant bearing on its effective delivery.

- *Patient-centeredness:*   Clinical teaching evolves around patients who form the basis of the 'content' of clinical teaching. The patient-specific discussion leads to development of general principles that can be applied to other similar situations. This is the most important attribute of clinical teaching and singularly distinguishes clinical teaching from topic- or subject-based teaching.

- *Encounter specificity:* Clinical teaching is mostly specific to a particular encounter and the discussion and teaching are directed to that encounter. The implication is that the learning cycle needs to be completed for each encounter and this may pose a significant challenge for the teacher and learner.

- *Unpredictability:* Unlike the other forms of teaching and learning experiences where the content and methods of teaching can be predetermined, clinical teaching is a rather episodic activity; there is little opportunity for continuity from one patient to another. Often the nature of patients' complaints or purpose of the visit is not known to the learner or the preceptor and the teaching has to be conducted without prior preparation.

- *Constraint of time:* One of the major challenges during clinical teaching is the limitation of time. This is especially true in teaching in the out-patient clinics where a typical encounter lasts for only about 15 minutes. The teacher is responsible to observe the students actively, assess their performance, provide feedback, and direct towards further learning. All these activities need to be completed within that stipulated time.

- *Clinical reasoning:* Clinical reasoning, the process of making decision about various aspects of disease and health of the patients, is an explicit goal of clinical teaching. Clinical teaching provides a certain degree of realism, ingenuity, and magnitude of patient data that are not easily available in other educational interactions. To promote clinical reasoning among the students, the teachers need to understand fundamental aspects of clinical reasoning process and target the instruction accordingly.

If we examine these factors critically, we realize that clinical teaching can be a very demanding task. The clinical teacher's or preceptor's chance of success very much depends on recognizing these challenges as well as understanding the learner's need quickly and efficiently and broadening the knowledge base of clinical teaching. Effective delivery of clinical teaching further improves with regular practice of a few selected 'skills' that specifically helps in situations where time constraint is acute.

Precepting in the Context of Clinical Teaching

Precepting is a *dyadic* educational interaction between the learner and the preceptor. The preceptor's role is to guide and train the learner in a way that gradually promotes the development of the beginners. As the precepting advances, the learner builds up self-confidence and trust to carry out the newly acquired skills or behavior independently and without supervision. In clinical teaching, the preceptor's role also broadens to include the role of clinical expert.

The physician, being the expert in the field, provides the requisite guidance that would groom the novice to become a competent physician. The success of this crucial transition depends on the interest of the expert preceptor in providing teaching and direction. The precepting process assumes that the teachers have some form of tangible or intangible interest in the success of the novice. In the absence of this interest the precepting process falters and the relationship does not mature to become meaningful.

The factors that promote the precepting process include mutual understanding between the expert and the novice, the willingness of the preceptor to provide the novice with space and opportunity to practice, validation of the novice's efforts, regular encouragement, and feedback. In clinical teaching, these translate into developing an insight into the present educational needs and expectations of the learners and helping to redefine the needs as necessary; a process that will be dealt with in the immediate next section.

Success in Precepting

- Expert's interest in novice's success
- Mutual trust and respect
- Opportunity and space for practice
- Validation and encouragement
- Feedback

Determining the Learners' Needs

As the success of precepting critically depends on identifying the learning needs of the learner, is there an easy way that would help us in the process? Let us broaden the precepting model and consider clinical teaching as a form of social interaction. In any social interaction, each individual approaches the interaction with a predetermined set of values and prior experience and expectations. The outcome of the interaction vastly improves with a systematic approach to understanding of these factors.

Similarly, during clinical teaching the teacher and the students come in contact with each other with a prior set of knowledge, experiences, and expectations. For the learners these determine the learning needs. But, it is erroneous to assume that learners know about their needs and deficiencies exactly. This lack of insight into their learning needs may not be necessarily limited to learners, as the preceptor may not be aware of the learners' needs and deficiencies as well. This creates a unique situation where learners may not know what they need to know and the preceptor may not know what the learners know. Based on these observations, we can devise four possible scenarios that may arise during interactions between the preceptor and learners (Whitman and Schwank, 1984).

The first situation is *shared knowledge* when the preceptor knows about the learners' knowledge. This is the knowledge and skills that the learners already possess. Nevertheless, the preceptor can further enhance the learning by way of reiteration, validation, and identification of key learning issues. The *hidden knowledge* exists when the preceptor does not know the learners' existing knowledge. The preceptor's role in such a situation is explorative; that is to determine the learners' prior experience, interest, and strengths. It is easier for the preceptor to prioritize the objectives and direction of the instruction with proper identification of hidden knowledge. The *known need* is what the preceptor knows about the lack in learners' knowledge and skills. *Unknown need* arises when neither the preceptor nor the learners are aware of the lack in the learners' knowledge and learning needs.

Therefore, the preceptor's role in effective delivery of clinical teaching is to explore the learners' preexisting knowledge and experience, and identify the known and unknown needs. The strategies for exploration include targeted questioning and review of the students' record. Educational interventions such as feedback, demonstration, and other forms of teaching aim to increase the shared knowledge and minimize the 'unknowns'.

Although the framework of social interaction is applicable for other learning situations, it is especially useful in clinical teaching because of the limitation of time and unpredictability. The challenge for the preceptor is to help learners learn the most important and most relevant topic in that short period of time.

Knowledge Base for Clinical Teaching

If we view clinical teaching as a form of social interaction between preceptor and learners with a defined educational goal that originates from and revolves around patients' problems, then the preceptor's roles, in addition to promotion of knowledge of the subject matter, include application of the knowledge within the broader context of the patients and their unique physical and psychological needs. The inculcation of such comprehensive knowledge and skills in the learners requires that the clinical teachers are knowledgeable in the subject matter as well other environmental and social contexts of their practice. The environmental and social aspects of practice that have important bearing on clinical teaching include knowledge about the demographics of the patient population, unique characteristics of the site, and prevalent nature of practice. The clinical teachers who possess these comprehensive knowledge bases are judged to be more effective.

The pioneering works of Irby and his co-researchers have identified the knowledge bases of successful clinical teachers (Irby, 1994). The following discussion summarizes the key findings from their studies.

- *Knowledge of the subject matter:* Effective clinical teachers have the requisite knowledge base of the subject matter. They are regarded by their peers and learners as erudite individuals. They are also able to reorganize and restructure the knowledge of the subject according to the needs of specific teaching purpose.
- *Knowledge of the context:* Effective clinical teachers possess insight and knowledge of the contexts about the patient and practice. Examples of such patient and practice related contextual knowledge include the nature of the patient population served by the hospital, the social characteristics of the patients, and the historical perspectives of therapeutics practices.
- *Knowledge of the patients:* The good clinical teachers should have elaborate understanding of the patient who is being discussed during clinical teaching. They should also have general knowledge about the patients served by the hospital.
- *Knowledge of the learners:* Effective teachers possess extensive knowledge about the learners. They are aware of the learners' needs and deficiencies and able to identify their strengths and misconceptions. Their experience allows them to anticipate in precise manner when, where, and what mistakes the learners are most likely to make and how to rectify the mistakes efficiently.

- *Knowledge of the general principles of teaching:* Effective clinical teachers are conversant with the general principles of the teaching and learning and able to capitalize on those principles. They regularly practice several effective teaching strategies such as active involvement of the learners, focusing attention to the specifics, broadening the scope of patient specific information, meeting individual needs, regular feedback, and assessment.
- *Knowledge of case-based teaching scripts:* Teaching scripts are short clinical vignettes that teachers are able to deliver within a few minutes. These are developed by repetitious teaching of similar cases. The teaching scripts contain internalized information about the goal of the session, key points to cover, specific instructions (e.g. analogies, examples, mini-lectures), common misconceptions and ways to address these. The teaching scripts help the teachers to anticipate learners' action in advance and enable them to respond quickly during the clinical teaching.

Thus, during clinical teaching the clinical teachers are engaged in two parallel and simultaneous processes. Firstly, the teachers assume the role of astute clinicians and listen to and assess the case presentation, interpretation of the data, and management plan by the learners. Secondly, they quickly identify learners' needs, anticipate their misconceptions, use selective teaching strategies to address these needs, and organize the session based on the learners' level of understanding.

Clinical teaching is a distinct form of educational activity with several important characteristics that have significant effects on the way teaching and learning should be conducted. As we develop greater understanding and appreciation of these unique characteristics we can develop more appropriate teaching strategies that specifically cater to the needs and demands of clinical teaching.

In summary, the important points that we have learned are

- The educational characteristics of clinical teaching include patient-centeredness, encounter-specificity, unpredictability, promotion of clinical reasoning, and time constraints
- Precepting is analogous to social interaction that benefits from recognizing the other party's needs and expectations
- The successful preceptor has an interest in the learners' success
- The effective clinical teachers possess comprehensive knowledge base that goes beyond the knowledge of the subject matter

References and Further Readings

1. Amin Z. Ambulatory Care Education. *Singapore Medical Journal.* 1999. 40(12): 760–3.
2. Hayes EF. Factors that Facilitate or Hinder Mentoring in the Preceptor-Student Relationship. *Clin Excell Nurse Pract.* 2001; 5(2): 111–8.
3. Irby DM. What Clinical Teacher in Medicine Needs to Know? *Academic Medicine.* 1994. 69(5): 333–42.
4. Knudson MP, Lawller FH, Zweig SC, Moreno CA, Hosokawa MC, and Blake RL. Analysis of Resident and Attending Physician Interaction in Family Medicine. *Journal of Family Practice.* 1989. 28: 705–9.
5. McGee SR, and Irby DM. Teaching in the Outpatient Clinic. *Journal of General Internal Medicine.* 1997. 12 (2 Supplement): S34–40.

18 Delivery of Clinical Teaching

A feature of medicine is that decisions have to taken frequently on the basis of uncertainty. ... Training in medical school is therefore expected to instill both the knowledge necessary to solve problems with clear cut answers and the capacity to reason and act in situations which do not have only one solution.

Benbassat and Cohen, 1982

In the earlier chapter, we have discussed several important concepts in clinical teaching including its educational characteristics, constraints, precepting models, identification of learners' needs and deficiencies, and the knowledge base for clinical teaching. In this chapter, we progress towards more practical aspects of clinical teaching and discuss how the concepts can be applied in real situations.

In this chapter, our tasks are to

- Learn about a useful model of conducting clinical teaching
- Discuss how clinical reasoning process can be taught effectively during clinical teaching
- Recognize the common mistakes that we make during clinical teaching

Models of Delivery of Clinical Teaching

We recognize that clinical teaching can be a potentially unplanned and chaotic activity. To compound the matter further there is a significant time limitation during clinical teaching which can be very acute in situations where the patient turnover is faster. For example, in out-patient clinics the typical time for a physician-patient encounter is 10–15 minutes. The actual time spent to deliver teaching can be as low as one minute per case (Knudson, 1989).

Thus, for clinical teaching to be effective within the limited time, it has to be highly organized and structured. At the same time it has to be based on sound educational principles. The learners' needs must be identified quickly and the instructions have to be targeted accordingly. Besides, the teachers' observations about the learners' presentation, clinical examination, clinical reasoning process, and management decisions have to be relayed back to the learners in the form of feedback. This vast array of seemingly unachievable tasks can be delivered with prior planning and with a certain degree of organization. There are several teaching models that can bring about the desired structure and effectiveness during clinical teaching.

One of the better-studied models is the 'microskill' model (Neher *et al*, 1992; Irby, 1992 & 1994; Gordon and Meyer, 1999; Furney *et al*, 2001). This is a step-wise and sequential model that progresses from diagnosing the learners' needs and deficiencies, teaching general rules, providing feedback by highlighting the learners' strengths and then correcting the mistakes. The following sections describe the microskill model based on their works with some modifications. We encourage the interested readers to read the original paper that is available on the web as well (Gordon and Meyer, 1999).

Five Steps in Microskill

- Step One: Get a commitment—ask learner to articulate his diagnosis or plan
- Step Two: Probe for supporting evidence—evaluate learners' knowledge and reasoning
- Step Three: Teach general rules—teach some general rules that can be used in future cases
- Step Four: Reinforce what was right—give positive feedback
- Step Five: Correct mistakes—provide constructive feedback with recommendations for future improvement

Adapted in part from Furney *et al.* Teaching the One Minute Preceptor: A Randomized Control Trial. *Journal of General Internal Medicine.* 2001. 16: 620–4.

Step one: Getting a commitment

This is the first step after the leaner has finished presenting the case. The preceptor's response is to prompt her to commit to a diagnosis or plan on her own. The cue often comes in the form of a short silence after the presentation when she expects some interference or guidance from the teacher. The teacher's response should be to resist making any preemptive comment and urge the learner to make a commitment. The rationale is that the process *diagnoses* the learners i.e. determines their learning needs and deficiencies. Without this proper diagnosis the learning is misdirected and valuable time is spent in discussing issues that the learner may already know or are irrelevant to their needs.

The questions that may help in this stage include:

- What are the likely possibilities in this patient?
- What is the most important piece of information you have obtained?
- What is the additional information you may want to know?

Step two: Probe for supporting evidences

Once the learner commits to a specific diagnosis or plan on her own, the next step is to probe for that assumption. The rationale is that it is worthwhile to explore the reasoning process in the learners' mind that leads to this assumption to identify the knowledge gap. The learner's usual response after making the earlier commitment is to seek validation from the teacher. The teacher's appropriate response is *not to offer any comment yet*, but probe for making the assumption.

The questions that may be asked in this stage are

- Why did you consider this as the most important diagnostic possibility?
- How is this information going to help you narrow down the diagnostic possibilities?

According to the precepting model that we have discussed in the earlier chapter, these two steps essentially target to identify learners' needs and deficiencies and reduce the boundary of unknown needs.

Step three: Teach general rule

Each patient is unique yet each provides a learning opportunity that can be applied to other patients' situations. The learner needs direction and guidance to connect the episode-specific learning experience to other situations with the help of some general principles. Teacher's responsibility is to teach some *transferable and reusable* rules about the patient that commensurate with the learner's level of understanding. The educational rationale is that instruction is easily remembered and transferred if offered as general principles.

Step four: Reinforce what was right

This is a form of positive feedback to the learner about the clinical encounters. The learners may not recognize the positive contribution that they have made during the teaching interaction or may underestimate the importance of their reasoning process. A good response by the learner may be out of pure luck and thereby easily forgotten. Reinforcement of such correct responses will improve the chance of permanent retention of the information. Providing positive feedback *before* correcting the mistakes preserves the learner's ego and self-respect and makes the next step more acceptable.

- You have considered 'A' as your first diagnosis based on the following reasons: ...Your reasoning process is correct because of these facts: ....

Step five: Correct mistakes

It is expected that the learners would make mistakes and wrong assumptions that might have impact on their future learning and patient care. If the mistakes are left unattended, they risk being repeated. The process of correcting mistakes is easier than it appears, as the learner may well be aware of the mistakes from the prior discussion and only needs reinforcement. The process becomes even more acceptable for the learners if they are allowed to correct themselves first. This is discussed in greater details in Chapters 15 and 16.

Thus, during clinical teaching this model progresses sequentially from identification of the learner's needs and deficiencies, then to provide general principles that are transferable, and finally to give feedback to the learner about her performance.

Teaching Clinical Reasoning Process

Clinical reasoning promotes critical thinking and problem-solving skills in the learner and is one of the major goals of clinical teaching. Teaching clinical reasoning process can be greatly enhanced from the understanding of the nature of reasoning process in clinical context and modifying and targeting the teaching accordingly.

Clinical reasoning is the process of making a series of inferences about the state of health or disease in the patients. The inferences are based on a multitude of patient data (history, physical examination findings, laboratory values, and therapeutic responses) and are interpreted in the light of existing knowledge and experience of the physician. An erudite physician is skilled in making connections between the apparently dis-jointed data. He is selective and efficient in data gathering, and able to make decisions with limited information, and proficient in recognizing patterns (Kassirer, 89).

Clinical reasoning usually follows several recognizable and overlapping patterns. We choose three common approaches to clinical reasoning and demonstrate how such reasoning process can be promoted during clinical teaching.

Probabilistic reasoning

This depends on determining the 'probability' of the event (e.g. likelihood of a disease, chances of successful treatment, and prognosis after the treatment) and is based on known prevalence of the disease and other statistical data. In an informal manner, probabilistic reasoning is exemplified by ubiquitous usage of qualifying terms such as 'likely', 'most likely', or 'rare'. More rigorous and desirable probabilistic reasoning thrives on critical examination of available data and application of that data to clinical reasoning. This method parallels the approach in 'evidence-based medicine.' Probabilistic reasoning may be exemplified by the question "What is the likelihood of vesico-ureteric reflux in a child with a first episode of urinary tract infection?"

The critical factor that determines the success of inculcating probabilistic reasoning among the learners is the formulation of *precise and answerable* clinical questions. Such question originates in the patient problems and should be answerable after reasonable efforts by the learners. This distinguishes itself from hypothetical questions or research questions that may not be of immediate relevance to patient care. The assessment of the reasoning process in this model depends on the *quality of the question* and *the process of finding the answer*. A good quality answer is desirable but not always necessary. What is of importance is the process the learners engage in while they search for the answers.

Casual reasoning

The casual reasoning process establishes relationships between two or more observed events. Thus, it examines whether the occurrence of event A can be explained by event B. This model relies on the understanding of physiologic, pathologic and therapeutic knowledge to explain the clinical event in the patients. Casual reasoning also narrows down the probable range of possibilities to a manageable few and categorizes them according to their importance. For example, during clinical teaching the learners may generate a wide range of diagnostic possibilities for a given patient's condition. The teaching strategy is to narrow down the possibilities by encouraging the learners to explain these possibilities in the light of known pathophysiological processes. This would eliminate those that cannot be explained while validating a few other plausible ones.

Frequently, during the process of casual reasoning, 'clinical models' are generated that comprehensively explain multiple clinical scenarios at the same time. Such a model is beneficial as they can be applied to other similar clinical situations with minor alterations and incorporation of a few other clinical variables. In other words, models help to create 'general rules'—a set of clinical dictum that is usable in other situations.

Deterministic reasoning

Deterministic reasoning is a categorical decision making model that depends on the generation of a set of clear unambiguous decision points. Frequently, such diagnostic reasoning evolves around 'if' and 'then' conditions that we set for a variety of clinical situations. For example, the statement "If a newborn baby presents with symptomatic hypoglycemia then the treatment is rapid administration of intravenous glucose," is based on deterministic reasoning as there is very little ambiguity about the action to be taken. More elaborately, deterministic reasoning model is encountered in the form of various clinical algorithms and flow charts.

Two factors are important during the teaching of deterministic clinical reasoning. First, the teachers should not only familiarize the students with the decision model, they should also *explain* the underlying reasoning for the decision. In the example of hypo-glycemia, clinical teaching should include an explanation of the ra-tionale for prompt administration of intravenous glucose. Secondly, the teachers should also emphasize possible ambiguous situations where such a deterministic approach is not practical or feasible.

Common Mistakes During Clinical Teaching

During clinical teaching even experienced and good teachers make mistakes. The mistakes follow a consistent pattern and may origi-nate anytime during the planning, teaching, and post-teaching re-flection phase (Pinksy and Irby, 1997). An experienced teacher is fully aware of his own vulnerability in making such mistakes. The factor that differentiates an effective teacher from a novice is the effective teacher's ability to learn from the mistakes. An effective teacher takes each teaching encounter as an opportunity to reflect and learn. He recognizes *failure is as important as success in the process of learning to be a good teacher* (Pinsky and Irby, 1997).

In the following table, there is a list of common mistakes that are recognized by distinguished clinical teachers during their own clin-ical teaching. Do we make similar mistakes? If yes, how frequent are they? How can we learn from these mistakes?

Mistakes During Clinical Teaching

- Misjudging the learners' strengths and weaknesses
- Lack of preparation
- Teaching too much content
- Lack of purpose in the session
- Inflexibility with teaching strategies
- Selecting wrong teaching strategies
- Inappropriately using certain strategies

Adopted in part from Pinsky and Irby, 1997

The other serious form of mistake that frequently occurs during clinical teaching is *overemphasizing unusual and esoteric aspects of patients or the disease processes* (Featherstone *et al*, 1984; Elstein, 1995). Physician educators tend to over-emphasize rare conditions ignoring the more plausible ones. During clinical teaching rare conditions tend to be over-represented, unusual anecdotes are used to bemuse the students, and there is a tendency to 'cover' even the distant possibilities.

Some of these are inevitable and may have reasonable pedagogical basis. Selective and judicial reference to anecdotes may be useful to highlight specific points during teaching, focus the attention of the learners to specific facts, and provide connection between the case in question and future cases. But indiscriminate and careless use of anecdotes and other clinical oddities jeopardizes learning during clinical interactions. The learners may possess immensely impressionable mind. They are easily gullible and tend to retain information in their memory for a long time even if the information is critically judged to be unsound. Unusual clinical cases or anecdotes have the potential for producing inaccurate and irrelevant impressions in the learners. Their use should be consciously curtailed during clinical teaching.

Although clinical teaching may appear to be a chaotic and unplanned activity, it is possible to render structure and organization to it to make the process effective. Many of the educational principles that we have discussed here are applicable to teaching and learning in general but they are remarkably helpful during clinical teaching.

In summary, we have learned that

- 'Microskill' model brings structure and logic in clinical teaching
- 'Microskill' sequentially progresses from identifying learner's needs, providing general principles, and rendering feedback
- Promotion of clinical reasoning is an important goal of clinical teaching

- Each of the clinical reasoning process requires somewhat different teaching strategies
- Unusual patient stories, anecdotes and other clinical oddities may actually harm the learning process

References and Further Readings

1. Benbassat J, and Cohen R. Clinical Instruction and Cognitive Development in Medical Students. *Lancet*. 1982. 9 (1) 8263: 95–7.
2. Elstein A. Clinical Reasoning in Medicine. In: *Clinical Reasoning in Health Professional*. Higgs J, Jones M (editors). 1995. Butterworth and Heinemann. Oxford. UK.
3. Featherstone HJ, Beitman BD, and Irby DM. Distorted Learning from Unusual Clinical Anecdotes. *Medical Education*. 1984. 18(3): 155–8.
4. Furney SL, Orsini AN, Orsetti KE, Stern DT, Gruppen LD, and Irby DM. Teaching the One Minute Preceptor: A Randomized Clinical Trial. *Journal of General Internal Medicine*. 2001. 16(9): 620–4.
5. Gordon K, and Meyer. Five Microskills for Clinical Teaching. Department of Family Medicine, University of Washington. Seattle. Washington. 1999. Web address: http://clerkship.fammed.washington.edu/teaching/Appendices/5Microskills.htm; accessed July 2002.
6. Irby DM. How Attending Physicians Make Insructional Decisions When Conducting Teaching Rounds. *Academic Medicine*. 1992. 67. 630–8.
7. Irby DM. Three Exemplary Models of Case-Base Teaching. *Academic Medicine*. 1994. 62(12): 947–53.
8. Kassirer JP. Diagnostic Reasoning. *Annals of Internal Medicine*. 1989. 110(11): 893–900.
9. Neher JO, Gordon KC, Meyer B, and Stevens NA. A Five-step 'Microskills' Model of Clinical Teaching. *Journal of the American Board of Family Practice*. 1992. 5. 419–24.
10. Pinsky LE, and Irby DM. "If at First You Don't Succeed": Using Failure to Improve Teaching. *Academic Medicine*. 1997. 72(11): 973–6.

19 Assessment of Clinical Competence

Assessment of clinical competency is a multifaceted process as this involves measurement of multiple and complex traits and behaviors that essentially include components of knowledge, skills, and attitudes (Carraccio *et al*, 2002).

In this chapter, our tasks are to

- Define clinical competency and related concepts
- Propose a framework for assessment of clinical competency
- Discuss criterion-referenced testing and its use in competency assessment

Concepts of Clinical Competency

The terms competency and clinical competency are used increasingly in medical education. Many definitions of clinical competency are proposed. Simply speaking, competency is 'the ability to carry out a set of tasks or a role adequately or effectively' (Burg and Lloyd). From the perspectives of education, competency denotes a trait different from knowledge acquisition and comprehension. Competency is more related to the ability of the learner to *apply* the knowledge and comprehension appropriately in relevant situations.

A related term is performance. Performance is defined as 'actual carrying out of the task or role' (Burg and Lloyd). Thus, although competency is a much valued attribute, it does not necessarily mean that the learner would *perform* the task in real situation. Further extension of the theme includes the concept of 'competent performer'—a learner who performs the task or the role in a competent manner.

In practical terms, a learner is considered to be competent if he is able to carry out a set of defined tasks that is considered by the professional body as a necessary requisite to function as an independent physician. Thus, a competent physician is able to provide medical care and/or other professional services in accord with practice standards established by members of the profession and in ways that conform to the expectations of the society (Whitcomb, 2002).

At a more micro level, competency is frequently used for a selected task or a group of tasks. Thus, a learner can be assessed to be competent for a specific task, such as endo-tracheal intubation, or for a specific role, such as an able diabetic counselor or for other intellectual processes such as problem solving and data interpretation.

Competency based education places greater emphasis on attainment of required competency and practice of skills in the real environment. It matters less how much time is spent and how the teaching and learning is being conducted. This represents a significant paradigm shift from the structure- and process-based models of medical education which define the training experience by exposure to specific contents for specified periods of time. A competency based education system, on the other hand, defines the desired outcome of training, the outcome drives the educational process (Carraccio *et al*, 2002).

Assessing Clinical Competence

Clinical competence is the end result of attainment of many

complex tasks and behaviors. Thus, during the assessment of clinical competence, students reactivate their past knowledge, elicit and analyze patient-related data, and carry out specific tasks. They are required to solve the problem embedded in the data and make the most appropriate clinical decision for patient's management.

The practical implication of these is that the assessment of clinical competence is unlikely to be achieved by a single test and there is a need to set up a *battery of tests* that would assess these intermingled parameters at the same time. Similarly, the assessment instruments have to be valid or authentic, resembling the actual tasks. Moreover, the assessment system has to be objective and there has to be sufficient build-in provision for formative assessment if necessary (Carraccio *et al*, 2002).

Elements of Competency Based Assessment

- Authentic assessment tools
- Multiple objective measures
- Direct observation
- Criterion-referenced evaluation
- Elements of formative assessment

Adopted in part after Carraccio *et al*, 2002

In the 70's, Harden introduced an assessment procedure, known as OSCE (Objective Structured Clinical Examination) that incorporates many of the above principles. OSCE has been accepted as a valid, reliable, and practical way of assessing clinical competence based on student's performance in history taking, physical examination, medical procedure, communication, data interpretation, laboratory test or X-rays. Clinical reasoning and problem-solving can be assessed as well (Harden and Gleeson, 1979).

OSCE has been used to assess clinical competence at the undergraduate and postgraduate levels (Kramer, 2002). It has also been used in licensing doctors in many places. More recently, OSCE has been validated as an efficient teaching tool (Brazeau, 2002).

The format of OSCE

In a typical format, the OSCE comprises several *stations*. In each station the students are asked to complete a specific task such as demonstration of a specific clinical examination skill, completion of a short written assessment or interpreting clinical or laboratory test results. Thus, the stations can be of two types: the 'procedure' station and the 'question' station (Harden and Gleeson, 1979). In the procedure station, students may be asked to do a specific physical examination or to take history of a patient with clinical symptom. In the question station, students have to answer multiple choice questions related to the interpretation of test results or management of the patient seen in the previous station. Each station is time-limited which is generally between 5 to 10 minutes.

Harden suggested a system of mark allocation that can be adapted according to specific training program:

- History taking   30%
- Physical examination   30%
- Laboratory test   20%
- Interpretation station 20%

An examiner is present at each procedure station where he observes and scores student's performance. He may also ask the student some questions to test his skills. In the question station the student answers on an answer sheet.

Possible Range of Competencies Assessed by OSCE (Harden and Glesson, 1979)

- Interpretation of patient's chart
- Interpretation of investigation tests
- Patient education
- Interpersonal skills
- Surgical or medical instruments
- Examination of specimens
- Examination of plastic models

Criterion-Based Assessment

> *The normal curve is a distribution most appropriate to chance and random activity. Education is a purposeful activity and we seek to have students learn what we would teach. Therefore, if we are effective, the distribution of grades will be anything but a normal curve. In fact, a normal curve is evidence of our failure to teach.*

Benjamin Bloom; questioning the logic of norm-referenced based curve in educational assessment

Once the data from the assessment test are generated, the learners need to be certified as competent or incompetent. Generally speaking, assessment data from educational measurements are analyzed and interpreted as either norm-referenced or criterion-referenced based format. We put forward an argument that criterion-referenced based format is more applicable to competency assessment.

Norm-referenced testing is based on the assumption that the score of a test result in a given student population follows a *normal distribution* (for example: the blood pressure profile in a community). The passing level and grades are pre-determined. Commonly, such levels and grades are either arbitrarily set or derived from the prior performance profile of the student population.

The criticism for norm-referenced testing is that this type of testing often compares one student's general level of competence with that of the others. In other words, norm-referenced testing doesn't factor each individual student's specific capability or achievement against the stated criteria. There is always a chance that a particular student will be judged as excellent if the rest of his peers happen to be poor students. Similarly, a student may be judged unfavorably even if his performance is of acceptable level when his peers happen to be of superior quality.

In the assessment of clinical competency, such approach of comparison of one's performance over the others and deciding the grades are obviously at fault as the crucial question is whether the individual learner has attained a minimum level of competency. Learners have to meet certain minimum criteria before being judged as professionally competent and not by mere comparison with others.

Criterion-based test is based on clearly defined test goals and standards of performance in the test. The strength and the weakness of a particular student are based on the proportion of those preset criteria that has been successfully met. The predetermination of the performance standard vastly improves the test validity (Calhoun, 86).

In summary, the key points that we have learned are

- Competency is the individual ability to carry out a particular task
- Clinical competency involves amalgamation of many different traits and abilities
- The assessment of clinical competency includes multiple objective tests, valid tools, and direct observation
- Criterion-referenced is the preferred way of interpretation of data from competency assessment

References and Further Readings

1. Brazeau C, and Crosson J. Changing an Existing OSCE to a Teaching Tool: The Making of a Teaching OSCE. *Academic Medicine*. 2002. 77 (9): 932.
2. Burg FD, and Lloyd JS. Definitions of Competence: A Conceptual Framework. In: *Evaluating the Skills of Medical Specialists*. American Society for Medical Specialties.
3. Calhoun JG, Ten Haken JD, DaRosa D, and Zelenock GB. Evaluating Performance in Surgical Education. In: *Medical Education: A Surgical Perspective*. Edited by Barlett RH, Zelenock GB, Strodel WE, Harper ML, Turcotte JG. Lewis Publishers, Inc. 1986. Chelsea, Michigan.
4. Carraccio C, Wolfsthal SD, Englander R, Ferentz K, and Martin

C. Shifting Paradigms: From Flexner to Competencies. *Academic Medicine*. 2002. 77(5): 361–67.

5. Harden RM, and Gleeson FA. Assessment of Clinical Competence Using an Objective Structured Clinical Examination (OSCE). *Medical Education*. 1979. 13: 41–54.

6. Harden RM. Editorial 2: Assessment of Clinical Competence and the OSCE. *Medical Teacher*. 1986. 8 (3): 203–205.

7. Harden RM. Twelve Tips in Organizing an Objective Structured Clinical Examination (OSCE). *Medical Teacher*. 1990, 12 (3): 259–264.

8. Kramer AW, Zyuithoff JJ, and Dusman H *et al*. Predictive Value of a Written Knowledge Test of Skills for an OSCE in Postgraduate Training for General Practice. *Medical Education*. 2002. 36 (9): 812–819.

9. Whitcomb ME. Competency-Based Graduate Medical Education? Of Course! But How Should Competency Be Assessed. (Editorial). *Academic Medicine*. 2002. 77(5): 359–60.

20 Teaching Procedural Skills

Clinical teachers are frequently required to demonstrate and teach procedures to medical students and junior doctors. Generally, such teaching is done without much forethought and incorporation of educational principles. Procedural skill teaching can be modeled upon sound educational principles to make the process more meaningful and effective.

In this chapter, our tasks are to

- Discuss the educational principles of procedural skill teaching
- Classify procedures according to the requirements of the program and student
- Justify reasons for abandoning multitude of obsolete ways of teaching procedures
- Discuss various effective methods of teaching procedures and analyze their rationale
- Identify the barriers to teaching procedural skills and ways to overcome those barriers

Teaching Scenario: You are precepting a group of house officers in the emergency room. This is their orientation week. Your task is to teach them airway intubation in a safe and efficient manner. You recognize this skill is very important for the learners to master. You also want them to build a sound understanding of the knowledge component of the skill. Accordingly, you have decided the goal of the session; the house officers should recognize the indications, contraindications, and necessary precautions of the procedure and they should be able to perform intubation in a competent manner.

Educational Principles

According to the American Board of Internal Medicine a procedural skill is 'the learned manual skills necessary to perform diagnostic and therapeutic procedures within the domain of the [internist]' (Bensen, 1984). Procedural skills are not unique to surgical specialties only; they are of immediate interest to most branches of medicine. Procedures are commonly practiced in ambulatory care sites, emergency rooms, pediatrics and internal medicine and other surgical and non-surgical disciplines.

The complexity and scope of procedural skills range from simple procedures such as laceration repair and lumbar puncture to more complex and comprehensive procedures such as surgical operations. Although the basic principles of teaching procedural skills are applicable to procedures with all levels of complexity, the average clinician-educator is more concerned about teaching commonly encountered and relatively simple procedures to medical students. We will concentrate our discussion on teaching these commonly performed procedures.

Conceptually, the procedural skills belong to the psychomotor domain in Bloom's classification. In reality, the skills required to perform procedures are complex and involve knowledge, attitude as well as psychomotor skills. In clinical medicine, knowledge is an absolute prerequisite to performing procedures in a safe and effective manner. Similarly, attitude and behavior are key components of procedural skills as well. These affective components primarily involve communicating with the patient about the nature, needs, and potential risks of the procedures, and understanding of and empathy to patient's problems. Although, the relative importance between knowledge, attitude, and skill varies depending on the nature of the procedures and the patients' contexts, all three are important to teach and learn.

Broad Categories of Procedural Skills

The number of procedures that are performed in medicine has increased dramatically with rapid advancement of medical science. Not surprisingly, physicians face the dilemma in deciding which procedures to teach and which are the priorities. Perhaps even more important is to decide which procedures *not* to teach to a given group of learners. Generally, such decisions are already made by the Faculty or certifying authorities who also determine the minimum number of procedures for the medical students to learn.

It is convenient to classify the procedures into three broad categories: (a) essential, (b) elective, and (c) not required, not recommended based on the demand and requirement of a given specialty and teaching and learning needs of the learners.

Essential procedures include both commonly encountered procedures (e.g. intravenous line insertion, lumbar puncture) as well as critical life saving procedures (e.g. cardio-pulmonary resuscitation). These are the procedures that every learner should be able to perform flawlessly and competently.

The nature of elective procedures varies depending on the curricular goals of the program for the given group of learners and available human and material resources. The number of procedures in elective category has increased parallel to the rapid rise in the number of procedures and tendency towards specialization.

Procedures which are not required and not recommended are deemed to be not suitable and/or not safe enough to teach and learn to the given group of learners. This again depends on the program goals, specialty requirements, and needs of the learners. For example, most programs do not allow renal biopsy to be performed by medical students, although this procedure may be considered as an elective skill for doctors pursuing career in internal medicine.

Less Desirable Way of Teaching Procedural Skill

Before we begin our discussion on sound methods of teaching procedures in the next section, it would be useful to revisit some of the older and near-obsolete methods of teaching procedures in medical science. The widely condemned 'trial and error' method appears to directly contradict the age-old guiding adage of medicine—'do no harm'. While as a clinician and educator we may not have any objection to supervised trial, we should question seriously the justification of 'error' that puts the patients at jeopardy. The other popular method 'see one, do one and teach one', appears to be more appealing, but there is a serious concern that such an approach results in passing inaccurate information and skills from one group of trainees to the next (Powers and Draeger, 1992). Finally, the concept of 'natural evolution' of psychomotor skills has never been substantiated by research. Procedural skills, like many other aspects of medicine, require active learning and training and do not result from passive evolution. Thus, even trainees from highly reputed programs may fail miserably in performing procedural skills if they are not properly trained (Wigton and Steinmann, 1984).

Structured Approach to Procedural Skill Teaching

The failure of the above methods calls for more scientific methods that are built on sound educational principles and are easily applicable. The idea is to teach and learn procedural skills in a more structured and effective manner without compromising patients' safety. It is also recognized that such teaching and learning methods should not be time consuming and should be easy to implement by a busy clinician.

Fragmentation of the main procedures into component parts

Sometimes procedures are complex and present with formidable challenges for the students and the teachers. The students feel overwhelmed by the complexities and are not able to follow all the steps in correct sequence and with acceptable standards. In such scenarios, it is useful to separate the principal procedure into component parts and allow the students to master one step at a time before progressing to the next stage.

The fragmentation of complex skills into component parts is often referred to as sub-skills or micro-skills method and is practiced in other situations such as counseling and clinical teaching. This method has been used successfully by several clinician educators especially in office settings (Barrett, 1984).

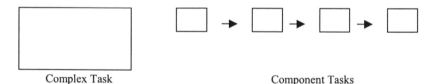

Complex Task   Component Tasks

The rationale for this approach is that complex procedural skills represent an aggregation of separate and discrete skills that, when combined in a proper sequence, collectively form the actual skills. These individual sub-skills represent varying degrees of difficulty for the students and may demand adaptation of multiple learning strategies. The students are more likely to succeed in performing the procedure if the main procedure is broken down into convenient small steps for them to understand and practice. When the students attain mastery of a specific step it bolsters their confidence and motivation to perform the subsequent steps. The sub-skills method is also convenient in teaching those technically complex procedures that the students may not need to master entirely. For these procedures, there are identifiable sub-skills that are still worthwhile for the students to learn.

As an example, airway intubation can be broken down into several component sub-skills: (a) recognition of the indications, (b) identification and arrangement of equipments, (c) safety precautions and monitoring, (d) positioning of the patient, (e) identification of the correct anatomy, (f) introduction of artificial airway, (g) ascertainment of the position of the tube, and (h) stabilization of the artificial airway. As the students become efficient in one step they are allowed to progress to the subsequent steps. Such a graded approach ensures that each step is done correctly and the students know the steps before moving to the next.

Teaching procedures as a whole but with lower levels of efficiency

In this approach, the procedure is preserved as a whole and taught and practiced without breaking down into component parts. The rationale is that the learners are not expected to master the skill entirely right from the onset. Thus, the expectation of accuracy of performance is lower at the beginning and with time and practice this becomes more demanding until the desired level of performance is demonstrated.

There are situations when keeping the wholeness of the procedures is important. Such situations may arise when it is critical to maintain the correct sequence of each step and the steps are too interrelated and dependent on preceding steps.

Teaching skills backward

In this method, the end result of the procedure is demonstrated and taught first. Such back-to-front approach allows visualization of the final product of the procedures. The approach is particularly useful when the learners lack sufficient motivation or are not sure of the needs of the procedures. Thus, in certain selected situations and with unmotivated students it may be worthwhile to demonstrate the last step first and progress backward (Robertson, 1980).

The obvious disadvantage of such a method is that the time requirement for mastery of the skills is much longer and it appears counterintuitive for the preceptor to follow and teach a procedure backward.

Another convenient framework of teaching procedural skills is based on the principles of taxonomy of educational objectives (Fig.1) (George and Doto, 2001). This sequential model emphasizes the learning of the cognitive component of the skills first (step 1). Subsequent steps include, in sequence, the preceptor demonstrating the procedure to the learners and narrating the descriptions of the steps involved (steps 2 and 3). In the final two steps (steps 4 and 5) the learners describe the procedure to the preceptor and perform the procedure under preceptor's observation. Table 1 details the steps, the rationale, and preceptor's and learners' role for each step.

Learners learn the cognitive components
↓
Preceptor demonstrates the procedure
↓
Preceptor narrates the procedure
↓
Learners describe the procedure
↓
Learners perform the procedure

Fig. 1. Educational taxonomy based model. (After George and Doto, 2001)

The choice of the methods depends largely on the students' needs and nature and complexity of procedures and has to be individualized. It is our personal preference to use sub-skills and educational taxonomy based methods for teaching procedural skills.

Table 1. A psychomotor domain based model (George and Doto, 2001) for teaching procedural skills.

Steps	Rationale	Preceptor's Task
Step One: Students master the cognitive components of the skills such as indications, contraindication, and precautions	Understanding the necessity of the skills motivates the learners	Teaches the knowledge components of the procedure
Step Two: Preceptor *demonstrates* the exact way the procedure is done without verbal descriptions	Learners develop visual impression of the procedure	Demonstrates procedure to the learners with or without the help of mannequins
Step Three: Preceptor repeats the procedure and *describes* each step	Learners' chance of success improves if they are able to narrate the procedure Allows learners to clarify their doubts	Repeats the procedure again Narrates the steps
Step Four: Learners sequentially *describe* the steps to the preceptor	Builds up the memory of the procedure Allows preceptor to correct the learner	Listens to the students describing the procedure Corrects and reinforces if necessary
Step Five: Learners *perform* the procedure	Learners are ready to demonstrate the procedure	Preceptor observes and provides feedback Allows the student to repeat the procedure until desired proficiency is achieved

Barriers to Learning and Teaching Procedural Skills

Many of the commonly encountered problems or barriers for teaching procedural skills are easily recognizable and correctable. If learners lack motivation it is most likely due to an incorrect perception or inadequacy of knowledge about the importance of the procedure. Proper knowledge build-up alleviates the problem. Sometimes, learners may have strong and long-lasting wrong images of a procedure in mind. Repeated reinforcement and feedback help the learners to erase the wrong images of the procedure and practice the correct one. Learners' trait inability refers to the inherent incapacity of the learners to perform a task. This may be due to a lack of proper neuromuscular or visual coordination (George and Doto, 2001). Recognizing the learners' limit of performance is crucial to preserve self-esteem and morale and to guide them to the directions where their chances of success are higher. Sometimes, learners face difficulty in transferring skills from practice to real-life situations. This is more likely to happen when practice or simulated situations are vastly different from actual scenarios where the skills are expected to be practiced. This is alleviated by practicing the skills in real situations (if feasible) or by graded transfer.

Barriers to Procedural Skill Teaching

- Lack of motivation
- Wrong images of the procedures
- Learners' inherent inability
- Difficulty of transferring the skills

Because procedural skills are a combination of cognitive (knowledge), motor, and affective domains, teaching procedures are intellectually challenging and stimulating. The methods that are described here initially may appear to be time-consuming and unsuitable for busy physicians. With repeated practice required time can be reduced to fit the teaching within the schedules. The time saved from correcting wrong procedural skills and satisfaction of preserving patients' safety are good enough reasons to teach procedural skills in an educationally sound manner.

In summary, we have learned that

- Procedural skills teaching involves comprehensive engagement of knowledge, attitude, and skill

- For teaching purposes, procedures are classified as (a) essential, (b) elective, and (c) not-required, not recommended
- Many conventional ways of teaching procedural skills are not scientifically sound
- Procedures can be taught in various ways depending upon the nature of procedures and students' own interest and ability
- Usual barriers for learning are lack of motivation, wrong image of the procedures, inherent inability, and difficulty of transferring skills to real situations

---

Tips on Teaching Procedural Skills

- Advance from known to unknown as new knowledge and skill are constructed upon pre-existing knowledge and skill
- Emphasize the knowledge and attitude component of skills
- Practice and teach safer aspects of the procedure first
- Allow learner sufficient time to be familiar with the equipments
- Determine the end points of the each procedure based on students' and programs' needs and requirements
- Be cognizant of learner's ability and needs

References and Further Readings

1. Barrett JA. A 'Subskills' Method for Teaching Surgical Skills. *Focus on Surgical Education*. Newsletter. 1984; 1–3.
2. Benson JA *et al*. Evaluation of Clinical Competence. Portland, Oregon. September. 1983. The American Board of Internal Medicine.
3. George JH, and Doto FX. A Simple Five Step Method for Teaching Procedural Skills. *Family Medicine*. 2001; 33(8): 577–8.
4. Powers LR, and Draeger SK. Using Workshop to Teach Residents Primary Care Procedures. *Academic Medicine*. 1992; 67(11): 743–5.

5. Robertson CM. *Clinical Teaching*. 1980. First Edition. Pitmann Medical. Kent. UK.
6. Wigton RS, and Steinmann WC. Procedural Skill Training in the Internal Medicine. *Journal of Medical Education*. 1984; 59: 392–400.

21 Teaching Communication Skills

Communication between the doctor and the patient is one of the key determinants of the patient-related outcomes in medicine. It is an essential component in the training of medical students that has been neglected in the past. Fortunately, this is changing with most leading medical schools incorporating formal communication skill training in their curriculum.

In this chapter, our tasks are to

- Highlight the importance of communication skill training
- Discuss the educational principles behind communication skill training
- Identify the important components of these skills
- Critically review examples of communication skill teaching in the curriculum

The Magnitude of Poor Communication in Medicine

Communication with patients is an integral part of the physician's daily activities. It is one of the key components that differentiate 'good' physicians from their lesser-loved peers. The onus is on the physician to be a good communicator. It is a general expectation that physicians themselves are responsible for communication with their patients and such responsibility cannot be delegated to others.

The magnitude of the problem in poor doctor-patient communication is well recognized. It has been estimated that over half of the time doctors fail to elicit patients' complaints and concerns (Strafield, 1981). Doctors also tend to vastly overestimate the time they spend with their patients (Makoul *et al*, 1995), and there is often disagreement between the patients and the doctors about the nature of principal problems.

Miscommunication with the patients is recognized as a cause of poor health-related outcomes in the patients. Poor communication results in non-compliance with the medications and prescribed regimen that directly contributes to unnecessary hospital admissions, additional visits to doctors, laboratory tests, and even increase in premature and avoidable morbidity and mortality. In the USA alone, the economical burden of non-adherence exceeds more than 100 billion dollars each year (Berg *et al*, 1993).

The quality of communication is also a major determinant of litigation and patient complaints against the care-provider. A study of malpractice deposition has identified communication problems in 70% of the cases (Beckman *et al*, 1994). Often times the intention to sue the doctors is present even *before* the occurrence of the bad outcome. Interestingly, but perhaps not surprisingly, the quality of medical care *per se* is poorly correlated with occurrence of lawsuits. The quality of treatment as judged by peer review is not different between never-sued versus frequently-sued doctors (Entman, 1994).

Effects of Good Communication

Just as bad communication results in poor outcomes in the patient, empirical evidences have shown repeatedly that good communication substantially improves many health outcomes and results in better doctor-patient relationships. Good communication directly improves *physical* parameters such as better blood pressure profile, pain control, symptom resolution, and improvement in overall health and functional status. The psychological benefits include, among others, anxiety resolution and better emotional health (Stewart, 1995).

Good communication also generates richer and more informative data. The better quality and greater quantity of the data improve the diagnostic accuracy. The social benefits of good communication are numerous and include better patient satisfaction, better *physician* satisfaction, and reduction of litigation and complaints about the physicians. At an individual learner level, the beneficial effects of improving communication skills are pronounced. As the learner develops better skills in communication he develops more positive attitudes and is more likely to become a willing communicator.

Teaching Communication in Conventional Ways

Unfortunately, there are very few structured instructional modules and sessions for teaching communication skills in medicine. Most medical students and physicians learn communication skills by a variety of *ad hoc*, unstructured, and informal activities. Often, the primary intention of these activities is not to teach communication but something else; communication skill teaching is seen as an added agenda of the session.

One of the common modalities of communication skill teaching is the observation of 'bedside manner' of the preceptor or the peers. None of these is evidence based and on rigorous examination fails to demonstrate noticeable effect in inculcating desirable skills in the learners.

The failure of the above modalities stems from many factors. Firstly, communication skill learning should be a structured educational activity that has to be supported by multi-modal instructional strategies (Kurtz, 1998). Observation or learning from one's own failure is only a part of this strategy. Secondly, the knowledge component of communication skills is grossly under-represented in these informal activities. Thirdly, although casual encounters between preceptors and students contribute to role-modeling, studies have shown that such learning is a slow and inefficient process. Moreover, there is a real danger of modeling wrong attitudes and skills. Finally, in the passive observation models, there is no chance for the learner to practice the learned skills and receive feedback from the preceptor.

The need for a well-structured and formalized module in communication skill is now well-recognized and strongly advocated by virtually all professional bodies including the Association of American Medical Colleges, the Liaison Committee on Medical Education, and the General Medical Council of the UK.

Communication is a Learnable Skill

There is increasing realization that teaching and learning communication is a *learnable and teachable skill*. This represents a significant paradigm shift in our prior thinking that communication represents a person's fixed behavior and attitude. Good communication is an inherent quality of the person and therefore good communicators are born and not trained. Current evidence proves that the earlier assumptions were wrong and that communication is a learnable skill. Such skills can and should be taught.

Proponents of the skill-based approach warn against using experience alone in teaching communication skills because 'experience alone can be a poor teacher in communication skills. That is, without guidance and reflection, experience tends to reinforce communication styles and habits regardless of whether they are good or bad.'

Educational Strategies for Teaching Communication Skills

Teaching and learning of successful communication skills involve simultaneous implementation of several educational strategies

(Kurtz, 1999). Such educational interventions are more likely to be successful if they are offered and built-in within the main curriculum rather than developed as an isolated module.

The *knowledge component* of communication skill teaching provides the learners with the essential theoretical and conceptual frameworks of communication. It helps the learners identify the problems associated with poor communication and demonstrates the many benefits of proper communication skills. Therefore, good knowledge component in communication skills is essential to motivate them in learning.

The knowledge or the cognitive components of communication skills deserves adequate attention. There are many practical ways to build-up the requisite knowledge including several simple instructional strategies such as didactic teaching and provision of reading materials.

The *demonstration* of communication skills is important as it highlights correct communication attitudes and behaviors to the learners. The learners can also benefit substantially by observing the less desirable ones. Besides, the learners should be shown examples of the actual physical set-up conducive of good communication, samples of recommended verbal language to use in communication, and desirable body languages. Examples of appropriate instructional strategies include demonstration of live encounter by way of one-way mirror, and video-taped encounters with actual or real patients, and case-studies.

Simulation and practice of specific skills in a safe and sheltered environment is of paramount importance in adopting desired skills. It is unrealistic to expect that learners would develop the right skills immediately after the observation. Therefore, learners need to practice freely and repeatedly in safe situations first. The specific instructional strategies that would allow practice in safe environment include role-play and dealing with simulated patients.

Self-assessment and reflection are powerful components of learning communication skills. Reflection is an active and deliberate process whereby learners critically think about a specific encounter to identify the mistakes that have been made and self-suggest future remedial measures. Communication skills teaching is relatively difficult and often a sensitive issue for preceptors as it entails changes in personal idiosyncrasies, modification of own attitudes and behaviors, and incorporation of new ones. Reflection and self-suggestion minimize embarrassments and unwillingness in the learners and increase the chances of success.

Presence of supportive role models allows continuous nurturing and ongoing modeling of the desired communication skills beyond the teaching sessions. Medical schools and hospitals act as a 'moral community' and exert significant influence on the learners (Sulmasy, 2000). The cultural and moral values including traits of physician-patient relationship are transferred to the students. Moreover, supportive faculty members can validate good communication skills, encourage and motivate the learners for continual improvement.

Assessment is an essential part of learning and regular assessment of communication skills may promote the importance of communication skills within the medical schools' curricula. Good assessment reports justify inclusion of such teaching modules in the curriculum, reward and motivate the faculty members who have contributed to the efforts, and prove the importance of teaching such skills.

Admittedly, assessment of communication skills is difficult and appropriate tools with good validity and reliability are yet to see widespread usages. The tools that have reasonable validity and reliability to assess communication skills include observation and standardized patient. Fellow medical students, nurses, or the faculty can be trained to become skilled observers. Standardized patients, if properly trained, in addition to being a good observer, can provide feedback to the learners as well.

In appendix A, there is an example of actual communication skills observation guide (Calgary-Cambridge Observation Guide; Kurtz *et al*, 1998) that incorporates educational strategies that are discussed here.

Teaching and training communication skills require development of comprehensive faculty development plan to educate and train faculty on specifics of communication skills. The goal of

Table 1. Specific strategies to teach effective communication skills. (Kurtz *et al*, 1998; Reynolds, 1994; Stewart *et al*, 1995)

Strategies	Educational Rationale and Justifications	Examples of Teaching Interventions
Knowledge dissemination	• Provide theoretical and conceptual frameworks • Identify perils of bad communication • Recognize the beneficial effects of good communication	• Didactics • Group work • Paper-case
Demonstration of communication skills	• Identify the good and bad forms of communication • Develop alternative skills • Build wider range of skills	• Live or video-taped encounters • Patient's feedback • Actual sample of verbal and body languages
Practice of specific skills	• Practice specific or component skills in supportive environment • Gradual transfer of skills	• Role-play • Simulated patient encounter
Feedback	• Reinforce right behaviors • Correct wrong behaviors • Suggest remedial measures	• Self-assessment • Feedback by facilitators, simulated patient, and peers
Reflection and self-suggestion	• Provide suggestion and motivation from within • Less likely to create resistance to change	• Structured session on reflection • Reflective journal • Encouragement and support for self-suggestion
Assessment of communication skills	• Demonstrate progress of the learners • Gather support for the teaching modules	• Observation by trained peers, faculty, and patients • Standardized patient

such faculty development is the creation of 'education community' (Reynolds, 1994) in which a core group of faculty explicitly spearheads the teaching of communication skills and other aspects of professional behaviors.

In summary, we have learned that

- Good physician-patient communication improves patient related outcomes and benefits physicians
- Communication is a learnable and teachable skill
- Observation of 'bedside manner' is an inefficient way of teaching communication skills
- Successful educational interventions require multi-pronged strategies including building up knowledge, demonstration, feedback, reflection, self-assessment, repeated practice in safe and simulated environment

References and Further Readings

1. Beckman HB, Markakis KM, Suchman AL, Frankel RM *et al*. The Doctor-Patient Relationship and Malpractice: Lessons from Plaintiff Depositions. *Archives of Internal Medicine*. 1994. 154: 1365–70.
2. Entman SS, Glass CA, Hickson GB, Githens PB, Whetten-Goldstein K, and Sloan F. The Relationship between Malpractice Claims History and Subsequent Obstetric Care. *JAMA*. 1994. 272(20): 1588–91.
3. Kurtz S, Silverman J, and Draper J. *Teaching and Learning Communication Skills in Medicine*. 1998. Radcliffe Medical Press. Oxon. UK.
4. Kurtz S, Laidlaw T, Makoul G, and Schnabl G. Medical Education Initiatives in Communication Skill. *Cancer Prevention and Control*. 1999. 3 (1): 37–45. Accessed through internet; Dalhousie Medical School. Web address: www.medicine.dal.ca/medcomm/strategies/article1.htm; accessed August 02.

5. Makoul G, Arnston P, and Scofield T. Health Promotion in Primary Care: Physician Patient Communication and Decision About Prescription Medications. *Social Science Medicine*. 1995. 41: 1241–54.
6. Levinson W. Physician-Patient Communication A Key to Malpractice Prevention. *JAMA*. 1994. 272:1619–20.
7. Reynolds PP. Reaffirming Professionalism Through the Education Community. *Annals of Internal Medicine*. 1994. 120: 609–14.
8. Stewart MA. Effective Physician-Patient Communication and Health Outcome: A Review. *Canadian Medical Association Journal*. 1995. 152 (9): 1423–33.
9. Stewart M, Brown JB, Weston WW, McWhinney IR, McWilliam CL, and Freeman TR. *Patient-Centered Medicine: Transforming the Clinical Method*. 1995. Sage Publications. Thousands Oak. CA. USA
10. Strafield B, Wray C, Hess K *et al.* The Influence of Patient-Practioners Agreement on the Outcome of Care. *American Journal of Public Health*. 1981. 71: 127–31.
11. Sulmasy DP. Should Medical Schools be Schools for Virtue? *Journal of General Internal Medicine*. 2000. 15: 514–6.

Section 8

Instructional Methodology: Problem-Based Learning

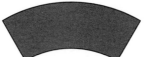

Assessment
and
evaluation

Educational
objectives

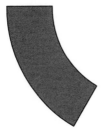 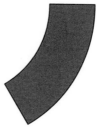

**Instructional
methodology**

22 Problem-Based Learning (PBL): Concepts and Rationale

True learning is based on discovery guided by mentoring rather than the transmission of knowledge.

John Dewey

In this first chapter on problem-based learning (PBL) we lay down the fundamental concepts and educational rationale of PBL.

Our tasks are to

- Define PBL in the context of medical education
- Discuss the historical evolution of PBL
- Elaborate on the educational rationale and benefits of PBL

Definition

The principal idea behind PBL is that the starting point for learning should be a problem, a query, or a puzzle that the learner wishes to solve.

D. J. Boud

PBL is an instructional method that challenges the students to 'learn to learn,' working cooperatively in groups to obtain solutions to real world problems (Dutch *et al*, 2001). The problems are used as a trigger factor to raise their curiosity and activate their prior learning. As such, the problem acts as an initiator of their learning. These problems simulate actual problems that are likely to be faced by the students in their professional life. Thus, the learning is *contextual*. Students engage in group activity and discovery learning and develop problem solving and critical thinking skills. Students also develop lifelong learning habits that include the ability to find and evaluate appropriate learning resources.

PBL differs from other problem-centered learning methods as in PBL the problem is presented *first* before the students develop substantial knowledge about the subjects. Typically, the PBL is introduced during the preliminary years (basic science years) in medical schools to integrate the basic and clinical science. As the problems in PBL are based on clinical scenario, they have a certain degree of realism and challenge by obscuring or 'hiding' the data from the learners.

The term PBL is used both as a curriculum option and a teaching and learning method. PBL as a curricular option replaces system-based or process-based curriculum as it emphasizes integration and consolidation by breaking down the artificial boundary between human body systems and subjects. In typical system-based approach, the curriculum is organized according to body system or functions such as cardio-vascular system or homeostasis function. Whereas, such separation is not present in PBL and a PBL case integrates learners' knowledge and enquiry in basic science, clinical science and preferably incorporates the psychosocial, moral, ethical, and legal aspects of medicine.

The perceived intellectual benefits of PBL are many and include problem definition, problem identification, data gathering, data interpretation, problem solving, critical analysis, and proposition of management plan. PBL cases are also believed to improve myriad of other traits such as communication skills, empathy, and altruism. Learners develop a 'broader perspective' of the case and acquire an ability to integrate psychosocial, ethical, and legal aspects of medicine.

Historical Overview

The inception and propagation of PBL in modern medical education is rightly credited to McMaster University Faculty of Health Sciences in Canada. PBL was first introduced in 1969. The factors that prompted the medical educators to take up such a revolutionary step were many. They were disillusioned with many ills of traditional medical curriculum, particularly the highly lecture-based and strictly discipline-oriented approach in medical education. They believed such approach hindered advance on medical education as the learner groups were passive, they failed to correlate basic science information during clinical years, and lacked the ability to transfer the learned knowledge into practice. The motivation of learning was external (clearing the hurdles of examination). There was little internal motivation and preparation for life-long learning.

Educational Rationale of PBL

The theoretical underpinnings of PBL are solidly grounded on several contemporary educational and psycho-behavioral theories. Albanese argued PBL process is supported by many theories such as information-processing theory, cooperative learning theories, self-determination theory, and control theory (Albanese, 2000).

For example, let us elaborate how the information-processing theory can be applied in PBL. Information-processing theory involves three major elements: prior knowledge activation, encoding specificity, and elaboration of knowledge (Albanese, 2000 and Schmidt, 1983). Prior knowledge activation refers to the concept that students use their prior knowledge and apply it to current situations to develop a new meaning to it. Encoding specificity emphasizes that learning is better if the learned materials closely resemble the situations where the learning will be applied. Finally, elaboration of knowledge means information will be better understood and remembered if there is an opportunity for expansion.

All the three components are actively practiced in PBL. The case activates the students' prior knowledge and provides opportunity to render a new meaning to it. The case also simulates the real-life situation and allows learning to take place in the context where it would be applied. Elaboration takes place in the form of discussion, question and answer that are expected of a PBL session (Albanese, 2001).

Objectives and Outcomes of PBL

For the Student

In PBL, students generate learning issues that guide their individual study. Students take an active role in generating learning issues, deciding how they will study them and evaluating what they have learned.

Benefits of PBL

- Problem-solving
- Self-directed learning
- Lifelong learning
- Resource identification and evaluation
- Critical reasoning
- Creative thinking
- Transfer of learning to real-life situation
- Incorporation of social and ethical aspects of medicine
- Cooperative and collaborative learning
- Group leadership and communication skills
- Identification of own strengths

Essentially, PBL promotes motivation, making students more engaged in learning because they feel ownership and empowerment of the solution development process. PBL also promotes metacognition (the skill of learning) and self-regulated learning. Students are required to decide on their own learning strategies during each phase of PBL process and compare with and share these strategies against fellow students' and mentors' strategies. PBL allows the learners to evaluate their own learning and adjust the learning strategy if necessary. PBL promotes reduced reliance on rote memory and greater reflection on the material they learn and how they learn it (Engel, 1991; Gwee, Lee, and Koh, 2001).

For the PBL tutor

PBL brings benefits to the tutors as well. The role of the tutors in PBL is vastly expanded, not contracted, to become a facilitator of learning. They are entrusted to motivate the students, nurture their learning process and model their behavior and thinking for the rest of their professional life. PBL provides excellent opportunities for tutors to build rapports with their students and become a partner in their learning. Tutors are required to learn about the many fundamental aspects of medical education that would not have been possible otherwise. Thus, they become more adept in tutoring skills and develop greater appreciations for active and interactive form of learning. Finally, non-expert tutors also broaden their own knowledge base and remain current with medical science.

Conclusion

PBL is a more holistic approach to education. Although it requires more comprehensive faulty development and training, PBL is more likely to meet the needs and demands of medical students, the profession, and society.

References and Further Readings

1. Albanese M. Problem-Based Learning: Why Curricula are Likely to Show Little Effects on Knowledge and Clinical Skills. *Medical Education*. 2000. 34: 729–38.

2. Albanese MA, and Mitchell S. Problem-Based Learning: A Review of Literature on Its Outcomes and Implementation Issues. *Academic Medicine*. 1993. 68 (1): 52–81.

3. Boud DJ. Problem-Based learning. In: *Education for the Profession*. Higher Education Research and Development Society of Australasia. Sydney. Australia.

4. Duch BJ, Groh SE, and Allen DE. *The Power of Problem-Based Learning*. 2001. Stylus: Sterling. VA.

5. Engel CE. Not Just a Method but a Way of Learning. In: The Challenge of Problem-Based Learning. Boud D. and Felletti G. Kogan Press. 1991.

6. Gwee M, Lee EH, and Koh DR. What is Problem-Based Learning? *SMA News*. April 2001; 33 (no 4): 6–7.

23 The PBL Process

Even if we are the only species that 'teaches deliberately' and 'out of the context of use', this does not mean that we should turn this evolutionary step into a fetish.

Bruner, 1996

In the earlier chapter, we recognized the PBL as a student-centered learning process where the teachers act as a facilitator. In this chapter, we advance our discussion on the practical aspects of PBL, especially its actual implementation.

Our tasks are to

- Discuss how PBL is practiced
- Discuss the essential features of various sessions in PBL

PBL is a method in which students are *first presented with a problem that triggers a learning process by discovery* (Barrows and Tamblyn, 1980). The responsibility of acquiring knowledge is 'given' to the students. Usually two to three small group discussion sessions of 2–3 hours each with a learning period of 4–7 days in between are allocated to each problem. In each group five to ten students work together with one or more tutors (facilitators). The small group session is known as tutorial. PBL sessions progress sequentially with meeting of the case-writer with the tutors, formation of the small group, and the tutorials.

Meeting with Case Writers

Typically, PBL cases are presented as a written patient case. The cases are developed by a group of case-writers who may or may not act as PBL tutor for the cases. Prior to PBL sessions with students, tutors are given the problem case along with a tutor guide and given opportunity to meet the case-writers.

The objectives of the meeting with the case-writers are several.

- To identify the learning issues of the case
- To provide case-writers' perspectives including the rationale of choosing the case
- To clarify obscure points in the case, if any
- Provide feedback to the case-writers on how to improve the case in future

The session is especially important for non-expert tutors as they have the opportunity to 'know' the case better. After the meeting with the case-writer, the tutors meet the students for actual PBL session.

Setting the Pace and Tone of the New Group

This important session sets the tone for the rest of the PBL tutorials by creating a comfortable setting that is conducive to learning. A properly functioning tutorial group rarely forms spontaneously. The group passes through a maturation phase before becoming fully functional (Chapter 12). The tutor plays a critical role in this formative phase and ensures creation of a group where learning is a spontaneous and pleasurable activity.

The tutor should adopt several strategies to create a proper functioning group. The tutor ensures that everyone is sitting in such a way that all members have eye contact with each other. There should be an introduction of group members revealing a little bit of personal information to get everyone into a more relaxed mood. If the tutor is not familiar with all the students, then he should either memorize everyone's names or get name-cards displayed.

Subsequently the tutor clarifies the roles of the students that include identification of the learning issues and learning resources. Then the students are reminded of their responsibilities for running the session. Students nominate a scribe for taking down notes on the board and another for keeping track of the learning issues generated. The students are also encouraged to designate individuals who will be responsible for following up on these issues in session two. The students are encouraged to nominate different people for these responsibilities at other sessions.

Strategies for Tutor During Small Group Formation

- Make sure everybody has eye-contact with each other
- Allow introduction of group members
- Address everybody by name
- Clarify the roles and responsibilities of the group members
- Assign a group leader and a scribe

Thus, the preferred atmosphere is an informal and relaxed one but not so much that it leads to somnambulism. Neither should the session be a 'free-for-all' where everyone is talking at the same time and no one is listening. Conversely, it should not be such that no one speaks up for fear of being ridiculed or having to ask permission from the tutor!

Session One

Session one heralds the actual start of work with the problem. There are six fundamental steps in working with a problem:

- Defining the problem
- Activating prior knowledge
- Brainstorming
- Generating hypotheses
- Formulating learning issues, and
- Identifying learning resources

Session one starts with the presentation of a clinical case where the current health status of a patient is described. The case preferably includes some patient pictures or records as well. Students then discuss and seek further information as necessary and try to clarify and define what the problem is. A medical dictionary should be available so that definitions of unfamiliar terms are agreed upon by the whole group.

As the students listen to the information given about the case, they activate prior knowledge and develop hypotheses to explain the problem. The group brainstorms by asking 'what', 'why' and 'how' types of questions. Each student should participate actively in proposing, defending, criticizing, and refining the hypotheses as more information about the case becomes available. As the list of possible hypotheses is generated, the students become aware of gaps in their pre-existing knowledge. This leads to formulation of learning issues relevant to the case. Therefore, the students decide what knowledge they already have and what else they need to know (learning issues) in order to clarify their understanding of the case presented. The tutor may intervene and make sure that all the important learning issues are covered.

At the end of session one, the students assign tasks to the group member to follow up on the learning issues generated. Then they identify learning resources that can be used to do so. These resources may include content experts such as doctors, scientists and others, and printed materials such as textbooks, published articles and reputable internet websites.

Therefore, in session one the essential elements are active discussion and analysis of the problem, generation of hypotheses on the mechanism(s) underlying the signs and symptoms, critical analysis of further knowledge required to understand the case, and identification of the resources for acquisition of such knowledge to be applied to the case in the second session.

Session Two

After a break of a few days when the students have obtained sufficient information on the learning issues identified in session one, the group reconvenes. In session two, there are three important tasks facing the students. First, the students determine the accuracy and validity of the information they have obtained. Thus, they review and discuss the effectiveness, appropriateness and quality of the resources they have used.

Secondly, they have to apply the new knowledge to the problem and integrate this new knowledge. So they review, share and evaluate their newly-acquired knowledge and information. They re-analyze the problem in the light of their new knowledge and where necessary, critique, refine and re-formulate their original hypotheses. They integrate and apply their new knowledge toward understanding the problem. They are encouraged to bring the knowledge that they have acquired in the form of published work, diagrams and/or notes and try to develop major concepts or principles that are relevant to the problem case.

Finally, the students complete an assessment of their own performance and the tutor's during the PBL sessions. Generally, the students self-assess themselves first followed by peer assessment. The group's responsibility also includes assessment of the tutor and the case.

In self-assessment, they need to be aware of gaps in their knowledge base, what they know, what they do not know and what they need to know. Peer assessment ensures the growth of the student within the group and emphasizes the cooperative nature of PBL. The tutor provides assessment or feedback that encourages students to explore different ideas, evaluate individual interaction in the group, and reflects the cognitive growth of the students. This last activity is important in allowing students and tutors to practice self and peer assessment as well as communication skills.

In summary, the most important points that we have learned are

- The PBL can be structured as (a) meeting with the case-writer, (b) helping to form a functioning group, and (c) working and resolution of the case
- Each of the sessions has defined objectives and tutors are responsible to ensure that these objectives are met
- Self-assessment and peer assessment within the group ensure sustainability and progressive growth of the group

References and Further Readings

1. Barrows HS, and Tamblyn RN. *Problem-Based Learning: An Approach to Medical Education.* Springer Publishers. New York. USA.
2. Bruner J. *The Culture of Education.* 1996. Harvard University Press. Cambridge, MA. USA.

24 The Tutor and the Case-Writer

[The PBL tutors] set the stage for learning and present themselves as models of the learning process. In so doing, they exercise an unprecedented and unparalleled influence on students. PBL sessions reflect the tutor's imagination, creativity, personality, and temperament. These sessions succeed or fail in direct proportion to the tutor's preparedness and training for the task, organizational abilities, interpersonal skills and sensitivity to students.

Mayo WP, Donnelly MB, Schwartz RW, 1995

The tutor's role in PBL is changed from that of someone who provides knowledge to that of helping the students to acquire knowledge, that is, from a teacher-centered to a learner-centered mode. Thus, a student-centered PBL session is one where the students play active roles. However, *this does not mean that the PBL session is a tutor-inactive one.*

In this chapter, our tasks are to

- Elaborate on the roles and responsibilities of PBL tutors
- Discuss the practical skills necessary to effectively run a PBL group
- Discuss the essential steps of PBL case writing

After completion of this chapter, we should be able to work effectively as PBL tutor and have the necessary knowledge and skills of writing suitable PBL cases.

The Tutor's Roles and Responsibilities

The role of the tutor during PBL session is multifaceted. He acts as a resource who is available to the students and also guides the students in the PBL process. He has to strike a balance between intervening too much, especially if he is a content expert, and thus undermining the students' self-confidence and the necessity to make comments or ask probing questions that guide the students in an active learning process. Thus, a tutor is a facilitator who encourages analysis, synthesis and evaluation of data. He encourages questioning and keeps the discussion focused on the problem. He also has to help in group assessment.

The characteristics of a good tutor can be viewed in three domains—knowledge, skills and attitude. In terms of knowledge, a good tutor should know the goals of the curriculum, the learning objectives of the module that he is tutoring in, the available learning resources, principles of assessment, and group dynamics. His set of skills should include facilitating learning, problem-solving, critical thinking, group dynamics or conflict resolution and assessment of the students individually and as a group. In order to be successful, the tutor should have the correct attitudes. He should be comfortable with the PBL philosophy and adopt a positive attitude toward PBL as a teaching method. He should shift his mindset from being a 'sage on centre stage' to the 'guide on the side'.

Just as we expect the students to develop and practice self-directed learning, the tutor needs to acknowledge that he does not know everything as well. As responsible educators, some PBL should be applied to the tutors too. So a tutor should try to learn more about the process and how to improve his tutoring skills which explains why you should read this chapter!

Unlike a lecturer, the PBL tutor's responsibilities now include being a facilitator, a resource person and the coordinator of the PBL sessions. As the tutor is a facilitator, he should not be dispensing information as an expert but again he should not just be a cheerleader. He should still have some authority within the group discussion but not be authoritarian. PBL should be seen as a cooperative session with reflection and critical discussion as part of the educational process. So, the tutor is not redundant. Rather, he is an integral and active but subtle participant in the PBL session.

Practical Skills

Intervening appropriately

When should an effective tutor intervene? He should do so to ensure that the students are approaching the problem in an appropriate manner and are not wandering too far from the learning objectives. He has to ensure that the students can clarify the assumptions and assertions they are making about the case. He should indicate any gaps in logic that are apparent. In intervening, the tutor should also tolerate wrong hypotheses suggested by the students as discovery, because wrong hypotheses are part of the active learning process that PBL is meant to encourage. Finally, he has to ensure that the students reflect on their performance as individuals and as a group during PBL sessions although this intervention should become less necessary as the group gains experience in the PBL process.

To be Effective, the Tutor Should Do the Followings

- Give up the role of the expert
- Intervene at appropriate times
- Facilitate the group discussion by asking probing questions
- Encourage brain-storming and problem-solving
- Foster critical thinking
- Encourage sharing of knowledge (without lecturing)
- Encourage student collaboration

- Foster communication skills
- Develop his own skills in self and group assessment

The Tutor Should *Not*

- Lecture
- Dominate the group discussion
- Act as a content-expert
- Be authoritarian

Asking probing questions

The effective tutor asks questions at the appropriate time and utilizes variety of questions and questioning techniques to help the group meet the objectives. In Chapter 15, we have a detailed discussion on question types and techniques; here we provide examples of questions that can be used during PBL.

Examples of Questions That Can be Used by the Tutors in PBL
Non-Directive Questions

- What is going on here?
- What do you mean?
- What do you think?
- Why do you say that?
- How do you know?

Directive Questions

- What other evidence exists?
- Is that a learning issue?

Directive But Non-Specific Questions

- What processes could have caused this problem?
- What are the mechanisms involved here?

The PBL Case-Writer

Profile and role

The case-writer is a very important part of the PBL team. He has to determine which cases to use to illustrate learning issues clearly so that the objectives can be achieved. Ideally, the case-writer is part of a team comprising a clinician with a basic scientist to ensure integration of the problems. The role of the case-writer is to prepare a problem with feedback from colleagues and other PBL tutors. He also has to prepare a tutor guide. After using the problem in a PBL session with students, the case-writer has to obtain feedback and improve further on the problem and tutor guide for the next batch of students and PBL tutors.

The PBL case

There are several characteristics of a good problem case. It should be at an appropriate level of complexity and at the same time refer to previous knowledge that the students already have. It should allow the students to achieve the learning objectives of the curriculum. The problem should lead to analysis and synthesis of previous knowledge with new knowledge.

Thus, the easiest problem to construct should be relating to a plausible common clinical situation. It should be motivating and interesting so that it encourages independent and lifelong learning. The problem should contain enough diagnostic materials and introduce basic principles of therapeutics. Overall, the problem must be written in a logical, clear, and concise manner. Wherever possible, normal reference values should be included when results of investigations are given.

The case should not require more than 90–120 minutes of discussion time during the two tutorial sessions and the interim self-learning period of a few days. There should also be minimum overlap with the lectures (if the PBL is part of a hybrid curriculum where lectures are also being given at the same time).

To make the case integrative it should highlight several issues or decisions which span and integrate various disciplines. It should link the basic and clinical sciences and raise social and ethical issues. The case should be interesting enough to trigger active learning. The students should be provoked into enquiry and discussion which motivate them to seek information and then internalize this information. Thus, a good case should be able to capture the interest of the students and tailored to the audience. There should be an element of puzzle, a surprise or emotional content. Multi-media or audio-visual descriptions could be used for illustration. There should be flexibility and freedom to learn within broad guidelines (the learning objectives should be given but remain flexible). The case should lead the students to formulate reasonable hypotheses and learning issues.

Characteristics of A Good Case

- Appropriate degree of complexity for the level of students
- Motivating and interesting
- Contains elements that refer to students' prior knowledge
- Leads to the students being able to fulfill the learning objectives of the course
- Leads to integration of basic and clinical science to the practice of medicine
- Well written, clear, and concise

The steps in writing a PBL case

In practical terms, the first step is to choose an appropriate case. To do this, the case-writer needs to look at the whole course schedule and the sequence of topics to be covered. Then he can choose several cases that cover one topic but which can be integrated with several disciplines. It is wise to have a few possibilities in order to create a bank of cases to avoid recycling the cases more frequently than once every three to four years. This way the students do not lose interest and of course, the senior students cannot then share case information with their juniors so readily.

The second step is to choose a good case that fulfills the learning/educational objectives of the course. Such a case usually demonstrates clinical features that the students are required to recognize and promote understanding of the scientific basis. Then, the case-writer starts gathering the necessary information such as case notes, laboratory test results, and radiology and pathology reports. The case includes enough data to make it interesting but not too much to confuse the students especially the younger ones who may get easily confused with redundant information. Modifications of the case may be necessary to make it interesting and to direct the students to fulfill certain course objectives. But modification should not jeopardize realism. Finally, it is always prudent to seek advice of the colleagues, especially those from other disciplines, to review the case for its clarity and ability to fulfill the objectives of the course.

The tutor guide

The case writer needs to prepare a tutor guide with additional information on the case and some sample probing questions together with the list of learning objectives that the case is trying to achieve. This guide is, as the title suggests, to help PBL tutor who are not content experts to facilitate the PBL sessions in a competent manner. Interestingly, many PBL tutors also find themselves learning from these guides.

This guide should contain the followings:

- Full description of the problem
- All the diagnostic materials
- Glossary for specific terminology
- The phenomena that need to be explained
- List of important concepts with short explanations
- The limits of the problem
- A list of possible questions
- A hypothesis scheme

The tutor guide may include issues that need to be avoided so that the students do not get distracted from the learning objectives for that particular case.

Reviewing and improving the case

Once a tutor guide is created, the case-writer should preview the case with all the tutors who will be facilitating that particular PBL to clarify any unclear sections. The experienced PBL tutors can tell if the case contains information that is misleading or is likely to confuse the students and how to make cases more interesting. After the case has been used with students, the case-writer should actively seek feedback from the tutors and students to improve the case for the next group of students.

Steps in Problem Writing

- Select a case that fits the curricular objectives
- Compile the necessary information (case notes, X-rays, laboratory test results)
- Prepare a tutor guide
- Consult colleagues for improvement of the case write-up
- Meet with all the tutors for a discussion and to make amendments if necessary
- Obtain feedback from the tutors and students
- Make necessary amendments before reusing the case

In summary, the important points that we have learned are

- The tutors play an active role in PBL by moderating, facilitating, and directing the group to achieve the learning objectives
- The practical skills of the tutors include judicious use of questions and questioning and recognizing the appropriate moments for interventions
- PBL cases should incorporate curricular goals and learning objectives

- Feedback from the students and tutors is essential for continuous improvement of the case

References and Further Readings

1. Mayo WP, Donnelly MB, and Schwartz RW. Characteristics of the Ideal Problem-Based Learning Tutor in Clinical Medicine. *Eval Health Prof.* 1995. 18 (2): 124–136.

25 Student Assessment in PBL

Elaborating an assessment plan that respects PBL principles, is reliable and valid, and has no negative steering effect remains a challenging task.

Nendez and Tekian, 1999

Student assessment in medical education, especially in the early years of the course, has relied almost exclusively on fact-oriented, multiple-choice or short-answer examinations. However, PBL is a process by which we expect the students to become a self-directed learner and efficient in learning, reasoning, and information-seeking. Student assessment should similarly be designed to reflect these traits and not merely for testing factual knowledge.

In this chapter, our tasks are to

- Discuss the goals of student assessment in PBL
- Propose a framework for student assessment in PBL

Goals of Student Assessment in PBL

The goals of student assessment in PBL are similar to the general goals of assessment but should be *aligned to the objectives of PBL*. Thus, the assessment system should provide feedback to both teachers and students on the degree to which the PBL objectives have been achieved. These methods should assess the skills that the student is expected to have learnt. Therefore, rather than just assessing mastery of content knowledge alone, the process skills of PBL such as problem identification, problem-solving and application of knowledge should be assessed. Finally, in the spirit of the self-directed learning approach, student assessment should be done both informally (frequently so as to enable prompt remedial action by the student/tutor) and formally (at the end of the course) in order to give the student feedback and more opportunities for improvement.

Special Objectives of Student Assessment in PBL

- Assessment of problem identification and problem-solving
- Provision of feedback to the students and tutors
- Application of knowledge into practical situations
- Contribution to group process

Assessment During Tutorial

An effective informal assessment of the contribution made by both students and tutors can be done at the end of the PBL sessions when the self-, peer- and tutor-led assessment can take place. Since these are informal, they are less threatening and there is a higher chance improvement. Less frequent formal assessment with a checklist or form can be made at the end of the semester/term. A sample of such an assessment form is shown at the end of the chapter. The form is designed to assess the student's attitudes and performance during tutorial sessions.

Objective Examinations

Content knowledge can still be assessed in the usual way by using various methods such as multiple-choice questions, modified essay questions, essays and others. OSCE can be designed to test clinical skills.

Assessing Process of PBL—Triple Jump

For assessing the individual's mastery of the PBL process, an assessment method called the "Triple Jump", as developed by the McMaster University, can be applied. Basically, this assessment method mimics PBL sessions except that the sessions are done by an individual student with the examiner/tutor.

In the triple jump, the student is given a case and asked to discuss with the tutor/examiner his hypotheses (based on his prior knowledge), analysis and other aspects of the case. Then the student has to identify and rank his learning issues. He is then given the opportunity to go away to obtain the information he requires for his learning issues. He then comes back and comments on what he has learnt to his tutor/examiner. He is required to refine his hypotheses in the light of his new knowledge and to critique his sources of information. Thus, the student is assessed for the skills that he is supposed to develop from attending the earlier PBL sessions.

In summary, the important points that we have learned are

- Student assessment in PBL should be aligned with the curricular goal
- Students should be assessed on those aspects of knowledge, behaviors, and skills that PBL is supposed to promote
- Besides content knowledge, emphasis should be placed on the students' ability to identify and solve problem, data gathering and interpretation, and application of knowledge in practical situations

- Students should be assessed on their contributions to group process as well

References and Further Readings

1. Nendez MR, and Tekian A. Assessment in Problem-Based Learning in Medical Schools: A Literature Review. *Teaching and Learning in Medicine*. 1999. 11: 323–43.

Assessment of Student by Tutor

Name of student: Name of tutor:

PBL Unit (s):   Date:

Please rate the following items according to the rating scale shown below:

1	2	3	4	5
Strongly Disagree				Strongly Agree

	1	2	3	4	5
A. Responsibility					
1. (S)he completed all assigned tasks to the level appropriate for the PBL session.	☐	☐	☐	☐	☐
2. (S)he participated actively in the PBL session.	☐	☐	☐	☐	☐
3. His/her behavior facilitated the learning of others.	☐	☐	☐	☐	☐
4. (S)he was punctual for each PBL session.	☐	☐	☐	☐	☐
B. Information Processing					
5. (S)he brought new information to the PBL session.	☐	☐	☐	☐	☐
6. The information (s)he brought in was relevant to the discussions.	☐	☐	☐	☐	☐
7. (S)he used a variety of sources to obtain information (textbooks, review articles, videos, etc.)	☐	☐	☐	☐	☐
8. (S)he was able to reason well.	☐	☐	☐	☐	☐
C. Communication					
9. (S)he was able to communicate his/her ideas clearly.	☐	☐	☐	☐	☐
D. Critical Analysis					
10. (S)he justified the comments (s)he made.	☐	☐	☐	☐	☐
11. His/her comments promoted understanding of the subject by the group.	☐	☐	☐	☐	☐
12. (S)he was able to think independently.	☐	☐	☐	☐	☐
E. Self-awareness					
13. (S)he is able to assess his/her own strengths and weaknesses.	☐	☐	☐	☐	☐
14. (S)he is able to accept and respond to criticism gracefully.	☐	☐	☐	☐	☐

Based on the above, his/her performance in the PBL sessions was

Below average ☐   Average ☐   Good ☐   Outstanding ☐

Other Comments:

26 Implementation Options of PBL

> *...each department is responsible for some part of the education of a medical student, but no department should forget that it is no more than a part of the whole school which is responsible for the education of a whole student and the fulfillment of the overall objectives.*
>
> Miller, 1961

We have explored what PBL is and the reasons for its wide adoption in medical curricula in many schools.

In this chapter, our focuses are to

- Discuss how and when PBL has been and is being introduced
- Discuss the advantages and drawbacks of some of the strategies
- Identify the factors responsible for the successful implementation of PBL

PBL in New Medical Schools

There is a wide variety of ways that PBL is being implemented. Obviously, if a new medical school is being established, it would be easier to have a complete curriculum that is presented in a PBL format. By this we mean that PBL is the way that the whole curriculum is delivered. The new leadership would use the same paradigms and share the vision that PBL is the preferred way to deliver medical education. Then new faculty can be recruited who are aware of, accept, and support the leadership's vision of the PBL curriculum. McMaster University in Canada and Maastricht University in the Netherlands are prominent examples of medical schools that have implemented PBL based curriculum at the outset.

PBL in Existing Medical Schools

However, not many medical schools have the above luxury. In existing medical schools, there are many constraints. Existing faculty may be resistant to the idea of giving up their role as conveyors of information and becoming facilitators of learning. Their mindset is still in a 'teacher-centered' rather than a 'learner-centered' mode of education. Financial, manpower and space shortages may also pose obstacles to the implementation of a full PBL based curriculum which can be demanding of such resources. Therefore, existing medical schools have used a couple of strategies to incorporate PBL into their curricula.

Parallel track

In the face of strong faculty resistance, one way is to set up a parallel track where PBL is used for a group of students at the same time as the traditional curriculum is being conducted for another group. Hopefully as the two groups are tracked for performance which can then show the superiority or at least the equivalence of the PBL curriculum; the faculty may then be convinced to convert over to a fully PBL curriculum. Of course, such an approach may lead to the staff appearing to put in more time into the 'new' PBL curriculum to the detriment of students in the traditional curriculum.

Pilot program

Another method that has been attempted in institutions with strong faculty resistance is to have a pilot program where just one course is taught in a PBL format. This has been implemented at the Otago Medical School in New Zealand with some success where the whole department of clinical biochemistry changed their curriculum to using PBL. Unfortunately, a pilot program in only one department or discipline can sometimes be unsuccessful because the students continue to be under a lot of time pressure from the rest of the non-PBL curriculum. They may not have enough time to explore PBL learning issues to greater and more satisfying depth. The successful planning and development of a pilot program or a parallel track need to be seriously studied so that the reasons for the success can be reproduced in other medical schools.

Complete shift to PBL curriculum

Very few medical schools have attempted to change completely from a traditional curriculum to PBL. One medical school that succeeded in this task is the John A Burns School of Medicine at the University of Hawaii. Here, the curriculum was converted to PBL in 15 months starting from the introduction of several faculty leaders to PBL and the planning and training of existing faculty to the full implementation of the PBL curriculum. The factors that contributed to this success have been identified. These include strong leadership of the Dean, successful choice of a consultant to guide the training of the faculty, involving all the senior administrators in the planning process and reorganization of the school such that all aspects of the curriculum became centralized and integrated throughout the course rather than being controlled by individual departments (Anderson, 1998).

In this model, there may be a short-term problem of the 'old' and 'new' curriculum co-existing for a few years until the students under the 'old' curriculum have graduated. For those few years, the students in the 'old' curriculum may feel disadvantaged as the faculty will spend more time in the implementation of the PBL curriculum.

Hybrid curriculum

Unfortunately, many medical schools do not have the luxury of running a parallel track nor a pilot experiment. For these, the compromise has been a 'hybrid' curriculum where PBL is used in parts of the curriculum simultaneously with more traditional curriculum. Many medical schools in Asia have opted for this approach where PBL is used as a teaching/learning method while reducing the number of but retaining traditional lectures, tutorials and laboratory sessions.

Advantages

The experience at the Harvard Medical School has shown that the hybrid curriculum can result in enhanced faculty and student enjoyment of the teaching and learning process (Armstrong, 1998). Faculty members reported enjoying all aspects of their tutoring experience from training with colleagues to working with students. Reviewing of the case-problems with the case-writers also provided opportunities for professional development. Students in the new hybrid curriculum showed no differences in their biomedical knowledge compared with the students in the traditional curriculum. However, the students in the new curriculum were better in their communication skills with patients and perceived their curriculum as more challenging, stimulating, difficult, and relevant. Some preliminary reports from a few Asian medical schools that have implemented a hybrid PBL curriculum have also reported similar experiences with their staffs.

Disadvantages

It is still premature to judge whether such an approach will work in terms of students actually reaping the full benefits of PBL in becoming more independent, self-directed learners. Theoretically, there are several disadvantages of such a hybrid curriculum, especially if the PBL portion does not appear to be assessed in an appropriate manner. Thus students who are only assessed on their content knowledge via examinations such as essays and MCQ will view PBL as secondary and only concentrate on acquiring knowledge in the traditional way. Moreover, if the lecture and PBL materials are overlapping, students may just use lecture materials when they are supposed to be looking for sources of information on their own during the PBL sessions, thus defeating the purpose of the PBL tutorials. The faculty may also slip back into their 'comfort zone' of being information-providers rather than facilitators. Thus, continual re-training may become necessary.

PBL in Asian Medical Schools: Issues, Challenges, and Options

A preliminary literature survey of the implementation of mainly hybrid PBL-traditional curricula in several medical schools in Asia has shown that they have adopted some characteristics that will allow these schools to address some of the problems that have emerged. Some of the reported difficulties in implementing PBL in these schools include poor participation and difficulty in getting students involved in discussions due possibly to their Asian reticence. One school reported that students felt that they were compelled to speak as they were being assessed. Some students reported not having enough confidence to seek information independently without guidance from their teachers. The students also found it very time-consuming to seek information themselves as they still had to cope with the requirements of the traditional curriculum of attending lectures. Some students had difficulty with the language if the PBL discussions were conducted in English as it was not their working language.

In order to overcome these difficulties, many of the schools realized that it would be prudent to start with careful planning and preparation with strong support from academic administrators. Otherwise, there will be a strong tendency for the faculty to point to these difficulties as evidence for the deficiencies of the PBL sessions. Furthermore, they will use these difficulties to argue for the supremacy of the traditional curriculum and lobby for a return to the traditional pedagogical methods.

Next, it is imperative that the students and faculty are given training and pertinent information on PBL. The trigger problems need to be designed carefully to make them relevant and interesting for the students. The language of discussion should also be one that both students and facilitators are comfortable with. Ongoing group monitoring and evaluation of the PBL process should then be incorporated into the implementation of the PBL curriculum. If these conditions are met, then the implementation of PBL should have a fair chance of success.

More Research

While we cannot deny the advantages that the graduates from PBL curricula seem to have, we are still not able to assess fully the graduates from hybrid curricula. There are many challenges and many questions to be answered. To what extent will PBL in a hybrid curriculum contribute to life-long learning? What is the best way to assess students who are in a hybrid curriculum? How can we know what is the optimal combination of different pedagogical methods that combine traditional teaching and more innovative learning methods? What are the strategies that will work best when we are trying to transform existing traditional curricula and incorporating PBL methods into them? How do we know when we have succeeded—that is, what do we use as the benchmark and the criteria for a successful hybrid program? We have more questions than we have answers. Thus, it is imperative that more research is conducted to try and address some of these concerns.

From the experiences of many medical schools, some criteria appear to be common to ensure successful implementation of PBL in medical curricula. These include:

- Careful planning and preparation with strong support from academic administrators

- Training of the teachers/tutors/facilitators *and* students
- Careful design of trigger problems to make them relevant and interesting
- Using language that the students are comfortable with
- Having non-threatening and comfortable surroundings for PBL sessions
- Incorporating on-going group monitoring and evaluation of the PBL process
- Using assessment methods that evaluate the skills obtained from the PBL process

References and Further Readings

1. Anderson AS. Conversion to Problem-Based Learning in 15 months. In: *The Challenge of Problem-Based Learning*. 1998. Second Edition (Boud D and Feletti GI eds), Kogan Page, London. UK.
2. Armstrong EG. A Hybrid Model of Problem-Based Learning. In: *The Challenge of Problem-Based Learning*. 1998. Second Edition (Boud D and Feletti GI eds). Kogan Page, London, UK.
3. Miller GE. The Objectives of Medical Education. In: *Teaching and Learning in Medical School*. Miller GE (editor). 1961. Harvard University Press. Cambridge, Massachusetts, USA.
4. Schwartz P. Persevering with Problem-Based Learning. In: *The Challenge of Problem-Based Learning*. 1998. Second Edition (Boud D and Feletti GI eds). Kogan Page. London, UK.

Section 9

Assessment and Evaluation

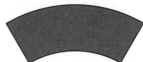

**Assessment
and
evaluation**

Educational
objectives

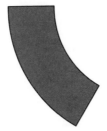

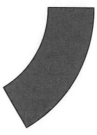

Instructional
methodology

27 Overview of Assessment and Evaluation

We should assess what we teach and teach what we assess.

Anonymous

With this section on assessment and evaluation we have reached the final phase of our learning cycle. This section deals with both formative and summative forms of assessment. Our primary focus will be student assessment, as this constitutes a very significant part of our educational activities as medical teachers.

The chapters within the section are organized as follows. The first chapter, 'Overview of Assessment and Evaluation', provides a bird's eye view of the topic and presents the essential concepts in brief. Some of these concepts are elaborated further in subsequent chapters. The second chapter discusses formative and summative assessment. The third chapter presents a detailed discussion on test characteristics including validity, reliability, and related concepts. The fourth chapter presents the road map to student assessment and discusses the factors that need to be considered in planning student assessment. This follows a series of chapters on individual student assessment techniques such as multiple choice questions, extended matching items, essay questions and their variations, oral examination, standardized patients, and portfolio. The final chapter discusses teaching program evaluation—a task that we are required to perform as well.

If you are familiar with the basic concepts of assessment and evaluation, you may read straightaway the chapters that interest you. Otherwise, we recommend that you start with the first four chapters.

Although in this section we principally discuss these instruments from assessment viewpoint, many of these instruments are *powerful teaching and learning tools* as well. Furthermore, almost all the summative assessment instruments can be used, with appropriate adjustment, for formative assessment.

Assessment and evaluation are critical steps in educational process. The key questions that are addressed in this phase are whether the learning objectives that are laid down at the first phase are met and more importantly, how the information obtained from the assessment and evaluation process can be utilized to improve the teaching and learning activities.

In this preliminary chapter, our tasks are to

- Discuss definitions and concepts of assessment and evaluation
- Highlight the broad purposes of student assessment
- Identify student assessment as a learning tool
- Determine the direction of student assessment

Concepts of Assessment and Evaluation

Assessment and evaluation are part and parcel of our daily activities. We compare, contrast, and make decision about various choices and options in life. During dinner or lunch, we compare one dish with the others and decide which one is the best for us. Although, this decision making process appears fairly straightforward, in reality it entails a comprehensive process that factors in many individual decision points—taste appeal, health needs, visual attractiveness, and affordability being among the major ones. Our prior experience and needs of that particular moment also contribute to the decision. The end result of these interconnecting and fairly complex algorithms is the decision about the worth of the dish.

Similarly, during teaching we constantly make decisions. Generally, these decisions fall into several categories; they may entail a *process* such as educational activities within a small group or the effectiveness of a lecture; or a *person* such as a student, fellow faculty member or myself; or a *program* such as an educational workshop or a course.

In medical education, process, person, and program evaluation are closely tied together. Moreover, the success of one may be the yardstick of success for the other. For example, the success of the course may well be linked to the success of students' performance. A pathology course may deem to be successful if the students' performance in pathology examination meets the expectation. In other situations, it is necessary to evaluate each component separately. For example, we may want to know what teaching strategy during the course resulted in superior performance of the students. Evaluation becomes far more systematic by identifying the most important and priority component of the evaluation process.

The questions that are of interest to us can be remarkably variable. For example, for the educational process during small group the relevant questions may be 'What are the activities that the students are embarking on to find solutions of the problem?' 'What is the quality of their efforts?' Similarly, when we are assessing persons the questions may vary. 'Who are the better students in this class?' 'Has this particular group of students achieved the necessary competency to be doctors?' Person focused assessment questions also include self-assessment. We may want to reflect back on our *own* teaching and judge its value. 'Have I reached the target of teaching?' 'Is there any room for further improvement?' Similarly, if we are conducting an educational workshop the important question might be 'Has this workshop attained the intended purposes?' 'Is this workshop worth the efforts and resources?' Common to all these is a *systematic data-based judgment.*

To give it a more formal tone, therefore, evaluation is the process of systematic data collection, analysis, and interpretation for the purpose of showing the value of a particular activity. More specifically, educational evaluation is a careful, rigorous examination of an educational curriculum, program, institution, organizational variables, or policy (Walberg and Haertel, 1990). For each of these categories, evaluation process may involve either understanding or improving the process already in existence—a formative evaluation. Or, the evaluation may entail passing a judgement of its intended or unintended outcomes—a summative evaluation. These two key concepts are elaborated on later chapters.

A related term is assessment. From the perspective of *student* assessment it is the process by which teachers judge whether the learning outcomes of the course are met. More comprehensive definitions of student assessment emphasize holistic approach and include '(a) systematic basis for making inferences about the learning and development of students. More specifically, assessment is the process of defining, selecting, designing, collecting, analyzing, interpreting, and using information to increase students' learning and development.' (Erwin, 1991). In program evaluation, data from the student assessment constitute only one of the many sets of data required to make a meaningful decision. The assessment data are considered along with other pieces of information such as program objectives and information about the teaching methods.

In this book, we have used the term assessment mainly to denote student assessment. The term evaluation is used mainly for program evaluation.

Value of Needs Assessment

Needs assessment is the starting point of good assessment that identifies the *current status* of the students or the program before the commencement of actual educational activities. Thus, needs assessment is used to determine the existing knowledge base, future needs, and priority areas that should be addressed. In this way, needs assessment can guide us to determine the areas that deserve greater attention and the extent of that attention. Furthermore, it allows development of a baseline to document progress of educational activities.

Basic Needs Assessment Questions

- What is the existing status of the students' knowledge?
- Do they already possess certain knowledge?
- What else do they need to know?
- What are the most important areas that we need to address?

Needs assessment can be conducted in a variety of ways. It may be done informally. For example, during clinical teaching, we may ask students the categories of common disease conditions they have not encountered yet. More elaborate needs assessment may include administration of a formal pre-test questionnaire and similar instruments.

Assessor and Assessment Audience

The person involved in the process of assessment is the *assessor*. The role, nature, and technical expertise of the assessor vary. Although most medical teachers are required to play the role of assessor, the more comprehensive assessment process often demands a level of expertise beyond the comfort level of ordinary medical teachers. Because of the complexity of the assessment process and the phenomenal importance of this in the educational process, many institutes engage specially trained experts. Frequently, they are educational psychologists and experts in educational measurement. They are not content expert, but collaboration between them and content experts (i.e. medical teachers) results in more meaningful and accurate assessment data.

The data obtained by the assessor are presented in a structured way that contains the findings of the assessment process as well as recommendations for its usage. This is an *assessment report*. The assessment report contains a large body of important data that should be properly utilized to improve the existing educational process. Any information of value, be it positive or negative; formative or summative, deserves proper attention. Thus, a good assessment report also recommends how the data generated from the assessment should be utilized.

Guidance for Utilization of Assessment Data

- Interpretation of assessment data
- Potential confounding factors and shortcomings
- Direction of their usage
- Potential beneficial effects
- Estimated extent of benefits

The assessment report also specifies who should be using the report i.e. the *audience* of the assessment process. The audience varies depending on the purpose and scope of the assessment and may include students, teachers, faculty administrators or professional bodies.

A good assessment report specifies the assessment audiences and caters the report to their needs. This crucial element ensures that the recommendations are carried out properly and more importantly, that the information is not misused or misinterpreted.

Assessment Audiences and Their Interests

Audiences	Questions That May Interest Them
Student	• How have I done in the examination? • How can I further improve myself?
Teacher	• How effective is the teaching module? • Is it adequate enough to meet the students' needs?
Professional Organization	• Has this student reached the required level of competency to perform as a physician?
Faculty Administrator	• Is the teaching program worth the resources spent? • Which one is the better performing teaching program?

Fundamental Steps in Assessment

- Decide on the broad purpose(s) of the assessment
- Focus on what are you assessing: program, student, or teaching method
- Choose instrument(s) based on the purpose
- Decide how the data will be presented
- Decide who should be the audience of the information
- Recommend how the information should be utilized

The Broad Purposes of Student Assessment

Principle 1: The Primary Purpose of Assessment is to Improve Student Learning
Principle 2: Assessment for Other Purposes Also Supports Student Learning

Principles and Indicators for Student Assessment
Systems, National Forum of Assessment

Why do we assess? What are the broad purposes of student assessment? The most important function of student assessment is to determine whether the learning objectives that are set *a priori* at the inception of program are met and to what extent. Student assessment also identifies areas of deficiencies in the student and educational program and suggests ways to correct those deficiencies. This way, another important function of student assessment, support of student learning, is fulfilled.

Support of student learning is often an explicitly stated objective during formative assessment and is widely accepted. It is easy to understand and be convinced about the role of formative assessment to support student learning. But how is summative assessment with its primary focus on certification and competency judgement linked with student learning? Is it a utopian concept? Is it really achievable?

To meet this goal, the educational objectives must be set after detailed consideration of *both* the educational needs as well as certification and competency requirements. If we formulate educational objectives in this way, learning and assessment become a closely linked coupled activity and both are achieved simultaneously.

A well-constructed assessment process generates a rich variety of data that can play a significant role in teaching program development and improvement. It provides information about actual program effectiveness, identifies the better performing ones, and points to mediocre ones. A good assessment also enlightens our knowledge about educational principles, processes, and theories.

The Broad Purposes of Student Assessment

- Determine whether the learning objectives are met
- Support of students' learning
- Certification and competency judgement
- Teaching program development and implementation
- Accountability
- Understanding the learning process

Directions in Student Assessment

As we have recognized earlier, the assessment is an integral component of overall educational activities and cannot be conducted in isolation. We have also identified that assessment aims to improve students' learning. Based on these philosophies, we propose several broad directions of student assessment that closely reflect the overall teaching and learning philosophies.

- *Assessment is driven by certification as well as learning needs*
  Assessment process should not be driven by the needs and requirements of the credential process and certification alone. Assessment should also take into account the learning needs of the students and be designed and utilized in such a way that it contributes to their learning.

- *Both formative and summative assessment are important*
  Assessment process should not be solely based on summative assessment. There should be fair and proportionate representation from both formative and summative assessment. Besides, good formative assessment is critical for successful summative assessment.
- *Knowledge, attitude, and skills—all should be assessed*
  Medical education comprises of knowledge, attitudes, and skills. Assessment process should test all three components of education and should not be limited to the assessment of knowledge only.
- *Emphasis should be on assessment of critical analysis and problem solving*
  Assessment of rote memory, although easy, severely constrains implementation of good educational models. As we promote and strive towards stimulating higher order cognitive abilities in our students, the assessment system should also test these abilities and not be limited to recall and rote memory.
- *All players should contribute to assessment*
  Assessment is not the exclusive domain of medical teachers. Students, medical educators, faculty, and professional bodies have important and legitimate interest in student assessment. Collaboration and participation among these different groups ensure that the assessment system remains credible and more reflective of their needs.

Current Status	Preferred Directions
Driven by certification needs	Driven by certification and learning needs
Based on summative assessment	Balanced contribution from formative and summative assessment
Assessment of knowledge only	Comprehensive assessment of knowledge, attitude, and skill
Assessment of recall of facts	Assessment of critical analysis and problem solving
Contribution from teachers only	Contribution from all players

Our aspirations are to create an assessment environment that is pedagogically sound, reflective of learners' and societal needs, and scientifically proven and reliable. We strongly believe an assessment system that strives towards these goals would also support a nurturing learning environment.

In summary, the important concepts that we have learned in this chapter are

- Assessment and evaluation is an integral component of learning; it is implemented in the context of overall learning and teaching activity
- Good quality assessment not only satisfies the needs of certification but also contributes to students' learning
- It enhances our teaching activities and provides valuable information about the educational processes
- There is a need to implement several changes to make the assessment process more meaningful and in tune with newer learning paradigms

References and Further Readings

1. Erwin TD. *Assessing Student Learning and Development.* 1991. Jossey-Bass. 14–19.
2. National Forum on Assessment. The Principles and Indicators of Student Assessment. Web address: http://www.fairtest.org/princind.htm; accessed on May, 02.
3. Scriven MI. The Nature of Evaluation. Part II: Training. 1990. ERIC Clearinghouse on Assessment and Evaluation Washington DC. *ERIC/AE Digest.* ERIC Identifier: ED435711: 1999-09-00.
4. Walberg HJ, and Haertel GD. (1990) (Eds.). *The International Encyclopedia of Educational Evaluation.* Pergamon. Oxford, England.

28 Formative and Summative Assessment

In this chapter, we further expand our discussion on formative and summative assessment—a pair of terms first introduced by Michael Scriven in 1967. Although these terms are used in different contexts and with different connotations, the distinction between these is often artificial and we regard these as complementary processes.

In this chapter, our tasks are to

- Describe formative and summative assessment as applied to the educational process
- Determine the relationship between these two
- Recognize how the information obtained from one process influences the other

Formative Assessment

Formative evaluation is a method of judging the worth of a program while the program activities are forming or happening. Formative evaluation focuses on the process.

Bhola, 1990

Formative assessment starts soon after the inception of the educational activities to either help learners achieve the learning goals and objectives or to identify the deficiencies in program's content and instructional processes. Data from the formative assessment are primarily used to further improve educational processes. Thus, this is a *process focused* assessment as opposed to outcome focused summative assessment. As such, it does not specifically seek to answer whether a particular student has achieved a certain level of competency or whether the overall program objectives have been attained.

In medical education formative assessment is carried out with several important predetermined objectives. Such objectives include assessing the learners as they progress through the course and collecting information to provide feedback. From the program's perspective, formative assessment is invaluable in determining the corrections and alternations needed in order to improve the program. Formative assessment also helps to determine the nature and extent of the required final assessment.

Therefore, both the learner and the program are investigated through formative assessment. The target audiences are usually the teachers or the organizers of the course and the learners.

Examples of formative assessment

- Providing feedback to the learners to determine their weaknesses and to improve their learning
- Conducting interim analysis of a workshop to identify deficient areas and suggest remedial measures
- Self-assessment by the students with reflection and self-discovery

Summative Assessment

> *Summative evaluation is a method of judging the worth of a program at the end of the program activities. The focus is on the outcome.*

> Bhola, 1990

Summative assessment is the most familiar form of assessment. The final exit examination in medical school is a summative assessment that certifies whether a particular student has reached the required level of competency to become a doctor. The commonly encountered questionnaire form distributed at the end of a workshop is another example of summative assessment. The common intentions are to ascertain whether the student has achieved the desired competency level or whether the program has accomplished its intended outcomes.

Thus, in contrast to formative assessment, summative assessment is *outcome driven* with the objective of documenting the achievements and worth of a student or program. Typically such assessment is carried out at the end of student posting or at the end of an educational program. Although, data from summative assessment are used to improve the upcoming educational activities, this is not the primary intention.

The major objectives of summative assessment are to

- Determine whether a student has achieved a certain level of efficiency
- Determine the extent to which original training objectives are met, i.e. to determine the worth of the program
- Compare between multiple educational activities and to choose the better performing one

For the students, summative assessment generally equates to course grades. For program organizers or policy-makers summative assessment is useful in deciding a program's worth or merit. Thus, it is often initiated and conducted by the decision-makers or by the external bodies.

As the summative assessment requires passing a judgement about the worth of some entity, the tone of summative assessment is much more formal and specific. The information is generally subject to more rigorous analysis and quality assurance.

Examples of summative assessment:

- Grading students at the end of the posting

- Collecting data on the impact of an educational program targeting the reduction of accidental falls from beds in the hospital
- Comparing lecture based teaching methods with interactive small group methods in a university in promoting learning

Traditionally, summative assessment has received more attention in medical education. We often erroneously tend to equate summative assessment with assessment in general, ignoring the rich role of formative assessment in educational processes. Good outcomes in summative assessment largely depend on the quality of formative assessment. A well-conducted formative assessment ensures that the student's performance continues to improve throughout the program and results in favorable outcomes during summative assessment (Fig. 1). Thus, it is strongly recommended to conduct both formative and summative assessment.

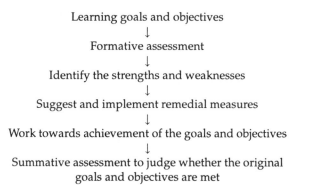

Fig. 1. The relationship between formative and summative assessment.

In summary, we have learned that

- Formative assessment is process-focused. It collects information from ongoing educational activities and feedbacks to further improve the learning and program effectiveness
- Summative assessment is outcome-focused. It documents the student's achievement or program's worthiness and frequently entails some value judgment

- These two processes are complementary to each other and data from formative assessment are vital for better outcomes during summative assessment

Table 1. Comparisons between formative and summative assessment.

Formative Assessment	Summative Assessment
Point of initiation is during the program	Point of initiation is generally at the end of program or at a predetermined time (e.g. mid-term examination)
Collects and feedbacks the strengths and weaknesses in order to improve	Records the achievements
Develops knowledge, attitudes, and skills	Records existing knowledge, attitudes, and skills
Guides and directs towards professional development	Summarizes the results of professional development
Generally recommended by the professional bodies	Required by the professional bodies

References and Further Readings

1. Bhola HS. Evaluating 'Literacy for Development' Projects, Programs and Campaigns: Evaluation Planning, Design and Implementation, and Utilization of Evaluation Results. Hamburg, Germany. 1990. UNESCO Institute for Education.
2. Wilkes M, and Bligh J. Evaluating Educational Interventions. *BMJ*. 1999. 318 (5) 1269–72.

29 Characteristics of Assessment Instruments

Assessment instruments have several important features that describe their applicability and utilities. The key terms that are used in the description are validity, reliability, objectivity, and practicability. These technical terms are in common usage and important in understanding the key concepts in student assessment.

In this chapter, our key focuses are to

- Discuss the concept of validity and reliability in the context of student assessment
- Identify common pitfalls in student assessment that make the assessment technique flawed

Validity

Validity refers to the extent to which an assessment instrument or a test measures what it intends to measure. For example, if the purpose is to test the diagnostic decision making ability of the students, the test should be constructed in such a way that it tests that particular ability. The test would be deemed to be of high validity if it measures that particular trait and of low validity if it tests less important issues such as recall of facts. Similarly, if the objective of a communication course is to assess student's interviewing skill, the instrument should be designed to measure that specific ability. An example of an assessment instrument with high validity to assess this skill is standardized patient. Conversely, a paper and pencil based test for this purpose is considered a low validity instrument as this measures content knowledge but not the interviewing skill of the student.

Thus, validity of a test item is *specific for the particular content area and for the specific purpose*. A test item that is highly valid in one situation may not be so in other situations. In the above example of communication course, the paper and pencil based test may be of certain validity if objective of the test is to assess solely student's content knowledge in communication. It is of low validity, as discussed, if objective of the test is to assess the interviewing skill.

Validity of a test item is not an inherent characteristic of the test instruments. It is a reflection of the results obtained by them and may depend on interpretation of the results by the examiners. The test instrument is valid if the results or answers obtained correlate highly with the intentions of the test. This is often a matter of judgement by the examiners or experts.

The concepts of validity are further expanded into content validity, construct validity, face validity, and predictive validity.

Content validity: This important concept refers to the fact that the test should assess the intended content of the course. Content validity ensures that knowledge and skills covered by the test items are representative of the larger domain of knowledge and skills covered in the course. For example, in a given course on infectious disease the goal is to test students' knowledge about HIV. It is not possible to test everything on such a broad topic. So, content experts or teachers determine what is important for students to know and the degree of representation from each area within the topic (Fig. 1). As MCQ-based examinations provide greater domain sampling, they can have higher content validity.

Construct validity: This refers to the compatibility between theory and methodology of the subject to be assessed and the type

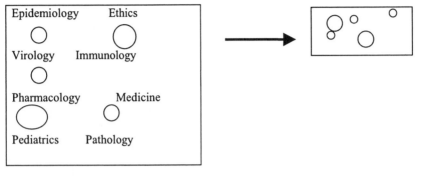

Core content covered in the course   Representative samples

Fig. 1. The concept of content validity.

of assessment. In other words, construct validity emphasizes that assessment techniques should be based on the nature of the content that they are supposed to measure. For example, a simulated patient-based examination to test doctor-patient communication skills has higher construct validity as it closely resembles the actual situation.

Predictive validity: This refers to what degree a test item for a particular content area predicts the students' performance or knowledge in another content area or in another situation. For example, we may want to know to what degree result obtained during a test of anatomy of nervous system predicts the performance of the students during clinical years in understanding clinical manifestations of cerebro-vascular accident.

Face validity: This denotes that the test item should appear to both students and examiners as though it measures what it is supposed to measure.

Reliability

Reliability refers to *consistency of test scores* and the concept of reliability is linked to specific types of consistency. Examples of how different types of consistency determine reliability include:

(a) Consistency of the results over time
(b) Consistency of the results between different examiners
(c) Consistency of the results with different testing conditions, including with different patients (i.e. classroom and patient's bedside)

Unlike validity, reliability is an inherent quality of a test item. Thus, internal characteristics of a test item either negatively or positively influence the reliability. For example, a clear unambiguous question improves reliability by generating consistent patterns of response from the students. Similarly, a longer test with multiple items is more likely to have better reliability than a shorter test with a limited number of items as the former 'evens out' possible inconsistencies of individual items.

The reliability of test items is a statistical concept and generally expressed numerically as reliability coefficient or standard error. Such as, there is 80% consistency (hence reliability) among the experts in identifying the correct response of this question. The measurement of reliability of test items is most commonly accomplished by establishing correlation by using test-retest over several time-frames, with different examiners, or with different testing conditions. Comparison with equivalent test forms is also helpful.

Objectivity

Objectivity of a test item is a similar concept to reliability. This refers to the degree of agreement between several unbiased and independent content-experts in choosing the correct answer. A question is high in objectivity if all or nearly all examiners agree to the correct answer. Conversely, if there is significant disagreement about the correct answer then the test item is considered to be low in objectivity.

Practicability

Practicability refers to the overall ease of construction, administration, scoring, and reporting of an assessment instrument. A highly valid assessment instrument may not be very practical to administer. For example, standardized patients provide practical advantages over real patients as they are more easily available and do not cause inconvenience to real patients.

Value

Value refers to the ability of assessment instruments to produce meaningful and usable information. An assessment method that is directly related to patient care is considered to be of high value.

Characteristics of Test Items

- Validity: The ability of the test to measure what it is supposed to measure.
- Reliability: The consistency of the test scores over time, under different testing conditions, and with different raters.
- Objectivity: The degree by which learned and independent examiners agree to the correct answer.
- Practicability: The easiness and feasibility of the test to administer.
- Value: The utility of the test results in producing meaningful conclusions about educational processes.

The relationship between validity and reliability is complex. A test item that is high in reliability may not be necessarily valid. For example, 'What is the commonest chromosomal abnormality in Down's syndrome?' is a question with a high degree of reliability with a standard answer. But if the focus of the test is to assess the core knowledge necessary for counseling the parents on the risk of recurrence of the disease in future pregnancies, then this question may not be high in validity. The students need to have some other additional knowledge beyond knowing that simple fact.

Nevertheless, a highly reliable test improves the validity and a test that is not reliable is likely to be low in validity. Reliability is thus a necessary but not the sole determinant of the question validity.

The relationship between validity, reliability (consistency) and objectivity, and practicability is more apparent in the following example.

Objective of the test: The students will be able to distinguish between the common causes of respiratory distress in a newborn baby.

Format of the Test	Validity	Reliability and Objectivity	Practicability
Practical Clinical Examination: Students observe a baby with respiratory distress and make possible diagnosis through history and physical examination	+++	++	+
Modified Essay Question: Students are given a paper case of a baby with respiratory distress and supplied with laboratory investigations and x-rays	++	++	+++
Multiple Choice Question: Students are tested with series of MCQ on their knowledge of the newborn with respiratory distress	+	+++	+++

Errors in Test Items

There are few other terms that are used primarily to describe the common mistakes in setting up test items.

Triviality: This is the situation when an assessment instrument overly emphasizes esoteric, irrelevant, and less important topic. A good assessment instrument tests all the important components with logical representation from different components.

Ambiguity: Ambiguity in question setting usually results from poor instructions, faulty grammatical construct, or confusing terminology. An ambiguous question forces the students to spend unnecessary time in deciphering the meaning of the question. Both oral and written forms of examinations are prone to ambiguity.

Unintended clue: This provides students leads as to the possible answers of the questions. Test-wise students can spot the embedded clue easily and answer without having the necessary knowledge.

Trap question: This intends to misguide the students to a specific answer of choice by the examiners. In addition to being low in validity, trap questions are notoriously low in reliability and objectivity.

Conservatism: This reflects personal prejudice, hidden bias, or idiosyncratic opinion of the examiners. Examiner usually has a fixed preference for a specific answer and tends to ignore all other plausible alternatives. The oral examination is particularly prone to conservatism.

Most of these faults in question setting can be avoided with proper training, careful attention to details, and conscious avoidance of personal idiosyncrasies and biases. As the examiners may not have the insight to these factors, it is vitally important to verify and solicit constructive critique from knowledgeable colleagues. More specifically, no summative assessment instrument should be used in the actual testing without independent verification and solicited review.

Ask Your Colleagues to Comment On

- Relevance of the questions for the goal of the program
- Relevance of the question for the students
- Overall interest of the question
- Ease of understanding the instructions
- Identifying and agreeing with the correct answer

Basic Qualities of a Good Assessment Instrument

- Based on the learning objectives
- Logical and balanced representation from the content areas
- Commensurate with learners' level of understanding
- Acceptable validity and reliability
- Practical to administer
- Free from technical flaws

In summary, the important points that we have learned are

- Validity is specific for the given content area. The two important components are content validity and construct validity
- Reliability is an inherent characteristic of test items
- Triviality, ambiguity, clue, trap questions, and conservatism compromise test quality and should be avoided

References and Further Readings

1. Gilbert J-J. *Educational Handbook for Health Personnel.* 1981. Revised Edition. WHO Offset Publication Number 35. World Health Organization. Geneva. Switzerland.
2. Calhoun JG, Ten Haken JD, DaRosa D, and Zelenock GB. Evaluating Performance in Surgical Education. In: *Medical Education: A Surgical Perspective.* Edited by Barlett RH, Zelenock GB, Strodel WE, Harper ML, Turcotte JG. Lewis Publishers, Inc. 1986. Chelsea, Michigan.

30 Road Map to Student Assessment

The planning for student assessment necessitates careful consideration of multiple important factors. In this chapter, we discuss these factors and propose a 'road map'—a constellation of major decision points in student assessment.

In this chapter, our tasks are to

- Analyze the critical steps in planning student assessment
- Propose a schemata for student assessment
- Identify the correct type(s) of assessment instrument for a given purpose

Student assessment is a comprehensive decision making process with many important implications beyond the measure of students' success. Student assessment is also related to program evaluation. It provides important data to determine the program effectiveness, improves the teaching program, and helps in developing educational concepts. Moreover, results from student assessment are often the principal indicator for program's success.

We take a systematic approach in analyzing the important factors to help us plan student assessment. This 'road map' provides a deeper insight into student assessment and directs towards identification of correct type(s) of assessment instrument for a given purpose.

Factor One: Educational Objectives or Domains

Three broad domains of education, knowledge (cognitive), skills (psychomotor), and attitude (affective) are important definers of a medical student's success. Any given assessment instrument generally emphasizes assessment of one domain over the others.

Instruments for knowledge assessment are more plentiful and widely available and enjoy a higher degree of familiarity than instruments that assess skills and attitudes.

Many of the important tasks in medicine comprise significant utilization of all three domains. Knowledge, attitudes and skills are frequently integrated and inter-related and their separation is artificial. For example, the task of diagnosis and treatment of a patient requires considerable contribution from all three domains. At the very basic level, it entails knowledge about the disease process, skills to perform clinical examination, and the right attitude to deal with the patient. Assessment of all three domains yields richer and more relevant information.

Unfortunately, in medical education there is an over-tendency to confine student assessment to knowledge only. Attitude and skill assessment or comprehensive assessment of all three domains is less commonly done. The commonly used essay question and multiple choice questions emphasize assessment of knowledge. Fortunately, there are other assessment instruments, such as OSCE and standardized patients, that can be designed to assess skills and attitudes in a representative and balanced way.

The key step is to clarify what is the most important domain that we need to assess in this group of students for the given task.

Knowledge is important but may not be sufficient for many tasks.

- What is the most important domain I am interested in assessing?
- Am I interested in assessing knowledge only?
- Is it important to assess attitudes and skills as well?
- Does the task involve one single domain or is it a combination of two or more domains?

Factor Two: Level of Knowledge

A major objective in medicine is the accurate and consistent application of scientific knowledge in the context of patients and practice. Application of learned knowledge into clinical practice is a gradual process. Miller suggested that 'clinical competence' follows a natural progression (Fig. 1). Briefly speaking, in the first stage students know about the knowledge (*knows*). This is followed by understanding of the knowledge (*knows how*). Subsequently, students demonstrate how the knowledge can be applied in a real situation (*shows how*). Finally, the student practices the knowledge in real life (*does*). (Miller, 1990).

Assessment instruments vary considerably in their ability to address these different levels. Some of the commonly used student assessment instruments are severely handicapped in assessing higher levels. For example, MCQ are best in assessing the level 'knows'. With careful attention MCQ can be used in assessing 'knows how' level as well. But MCQ do not assess the next two levels. Performance in real life can be assessed by direct patient related assessment strategies including portfolios or, in the case of physicians, patient's medical records. But portfolio based assessment is not suitable enough to assess 'knows' and 'knows how.'

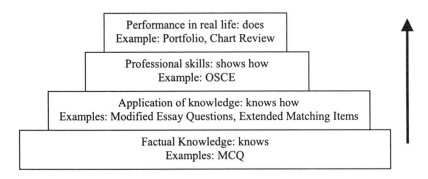

Factor Three: Formative or Summative Assessment

Deciding the purpose of the assessment, whether formative or summative, helps us to choose the right instrument. While the majority of assessment instruments can be used for both formative and summative assessment, they vary in their suitability.

Summative assessment is a formal process that often leads to certification or pass/fail judgement. The stakes are much higher in this form of assessment. Student assessment instruments that have a very high degree of reliability, consistency, and validity are better suited for summative assessment. For example, traditional oral examination is worthy as formative assessment, but lacks the requisite reliability and consistency to be a good summative assessment. Conversely, MCQ and structured essay questions are used for summative assessment because of their higher degree of reliability and validity.

Factor Four: Validity of the Instrument

Ideally student assessment should have a high degree of validity—it should be able to measure what we intend to measure. As validity of instruments is often specific to the domain, it is considered in the context of the main purpose of assessment. Realistically speaking, a high degree of validity, although desirable, may not be achievable for all instruments and a reasonable degree of compromise is often negotiated upon and practiced.

Factor Five: Reliability of the Instrument

Reliability is a statistical concept related to consistency of test score. A high degree of reliability is necessary especially for summative assessment. The instruments with high degree of reliability include MCQ, objective structured clinical examination, and structured essay questions. Reliability ensures transparency and fairness in the assessment system as well.

Factor Six: Single Instrument versus Multiple Instruments

It is virtually impossible to meet these different needs and purposes with a single instrument and to do so in an efficient and effective manner.

Roeber on the futility of single instrument based student assessment

We champion the holistic approach to medical education and aim to groom students who are not only knowledge-savvy but also proficient in skills and possess the right attitudes required by the profession. It is entirely justifiable and expected that the assessment system should reflect the philosophy as well. We strive towards an assessment system that assesses critical thinking of the students and pays due attention to other attributes.

The challenge is to assess medical students in accordance to the above philosophy. The recurrent theme that emerges from the above discussion is that there is no 'ideal' assessment instrument to fit all the purpose. All assessment instruments have their own strengths and weaknesses and are frequently useful for limited purposes only. Logically, medical schools frequently resort to selecting *a battery of assessment instruments* rather than relying on one single instrument. Each of the instruments fulfills specific purposes and caters to specific needs. They complement each other and provide a more comprehensive picture that would not have been possible with one single instrument.

Student assessment should not be limited to assessment of lower order cognitive domains such as recall and rote memory. Neither should student assessment be confined to assessing knowledge component. A variety of student assessment instruments are available that test different domains and different levels of application. Assessment instruments should be tailored to suit the needs of the programs including learning philosophies and objectives. Existing and well-familiar instruments can be improved and newer assessment instruments can be incorporated. There is no compelling reason to restrict ourselves to an insufficient number of student assessment instruments. We gain substantially from gradual exploration and incorporation of a wider range of student assessment instruments.

Our task in the next several chapters is to familiarize with several such instruments.

In summary, the cardinal points that we have learned in this chapter are

- The purpose of assessment should direct the choice of instruments. Availability, familiarity, and convenience of the instrument should not direct the purpose of the assessment
- Instruments that are highly recommended for one purpose may not necessarily be suitable for other purpose
- No single instrument has all the desired criteria; a reasonable compromise is needed and judgement has to be made
- Instruments for summative assessment should have a high degree of validity and reliability
- Multiple instruments provide a more comprehensive picture than any single instrument

Road Map to Student Assessment

- What is the domain I am interested in assessing?
  Knowledge   Attitude   Skill

- What is the level of competency?
  Knows   Knows how   Apply   Does

- What is the purpose of assessment?
  Formative   Summative

- What is the validity of the instrument for the intended purpose?
  Low   Medium   High

- What is the reliability of the instrument for the intended purpose?
  Low   Medium   High

- Is one instrument sufficient for the purpose?
  Yes   No

Range of Possible Instruments for Students Assessment

- Essay question
- Objective questions
- Oral examination
- Objective structured clinical examination
- Standardized and simulated patients
- Encounter with real patients
- Observations
- Video and audio recording
- Questionnaires and surveys
- Log Book
- Self-assessment
- Portfolio

References and Further Readings

1. Miller GE. The Assessment of Clinical Skills, Competence, Performance. *Academic Medicine.* 1990. 65: 563–7.
2. Roeber ED. How Should The Comprehensive Assessment System Be Designed? A. Top Down? B. Bottom Up? C. Both? D. Neither? In: *Evaluation Handbook.* Judith Wilde (Editor). Washington, DC: Council of Chief State School Officers. 1995.
3. Sockey S. Evaluation Assistance Center-Western Region, New Mexico Highlands University, Albuquerque, NM. Web address: http://www.ncbe.gwu.edu/miscpubs/eacwest/evalhbk.htm; accessed in May 02.

31 Multiple Choice Questions

Multiple choice questions (MCQ) are widely used in student assessment. The growing popularity of MCQ is in part due to its high degree of objectivity and ease in analysis and reporting. The construction of good quality MCQ to assess analysis, problem solving and other higher order cognitive abilities is a challenging but essential undertaking.

In this chapter, our tasks are to

- Identify the advantages and challenges of MCQ in student assessment
- Recognize situations where MCQ is an appropriate form of test
- Analyze how MCQ can be constructed following the hierarchical pattern of learning objectives
- Identify features of good MCQ
- Evaluate quality of MCQ by using difficulty and discriminatory indices

---

Road Map to Student Assessment

What does it assess?
Knowledge   Attitude   Skill

The level of knowledge
Knows   **Knows how**   Shows how   Does

Utility as summative assessment
Yes   No

Validity (content)
High   **Medium**   Low

Reliability
High   Medium   Low

Advantages

Well-constructed MCQ provide many advantages as an assessment instrument.

- *Broad content coverage:* MCQ can test wide range of topics of interests in a short period of time and in an efficient manner. The greater breadth and efficiency in domain sampling improves the content validity and provides significant advantage over other forms of assessment instrument.
- *Objectivity:* Good MCQ are objective—they are not affected by peripheral traits such as verbal or writing skills nor by examiners' preferences and idiosyncrasies.
- *Ease of analysis:* MCQ are easily marked. Good computer programs are available to optically mark items flawlessly and quickly.
- *Evaluation of test items:* MCQ can be analyzed before and after the test to determine their effectiveness.

- *Banking of items:* A large bank of MCQ can be created over the years. Individual item can be easily changed to introduce newer nuances of meanings and interpretations while maintaining the test confidentiality.
- *Transparency:* It is easy to provide clear, accurate information to the students about MCQ testing. Information about the examination such as format of questions, relative weightage assigned to each content area, time allotment, and grading criteria can be easily conveyed to students.

Limitations

MCQ have several disadvantages and limitations as an assessment instrument.

- *Assessment of knowledge only:* MCQ assess student *knowledge* of a specific content area. In situations where attitude and skill are important attributes, MCQ need to be supplemented by other student assessment instruments.
- *Restriction of choices:* MCQ are closed ranged questions. The students are forced to choose from the pre-selected choices that are provided to them. Utilization of Extended Matching Item (EMI) alleviates this problem. EMI is discussed separately in later part of the chapter.
- *Guessing:* This is a serious problem with poorly constructed MCQ. Many test-smart students are able to correctly answer just by deriving clues from the question.
- *Learning the techniques:* After several years of administering MCQ, students may become adept in recognizing patterns, clues and learn the techniques of answering MCQ without necessarily improving their content knowledge.
- *Possible negative effect on learning:* MCQ contain both correct and incorrect choices (usually more incorrect than correct choices). Students may develop more sustainable impression in their mind about incorrect choices and may remember those in future.

Poorly constructed MCQ tend to test knowledge recall and rote memory. MCQ that measure higher level cognitive functions are relatively difficult to construct. Examiners often resort to creating items that are easy to develop but fail to assess higher cognitive abilities. This is a challenge that is surmountable with proper training and practice.

Components of MCQ

A standard MCQ has a stem, a key, and several distracters. The *stem* is the opening statement that presents the problem. The *key* refers to the correct answer. *Distracters* are the wrong options in the MCQ.

Stem

The purpose of stem is to communicate the problem statement completely and succinctly to the students. It should not be too verbose and should not contain repetitious words and catch phrases. And for obvious reasons it should not contain clue for the answer.

Improvement of clarity in the stems

- Present problem as precisely as possible
- Ensure accuracy in grammar and sentence construction
- Use familiar words from the course consistently
- Avoid uncommon terminology and abbreviations
- Avoid double negatives
- Unless there is a specific pedagogical reason, avoid 'all of the above' and 'none of the above' options

Distracters

Distracters are the options that divert unsure students from the correct answer. All the distracters should be uniform and the correct response and the distracters should appear the same. The uniformity is achieved by ensuring that all the options are of (a) same length, (b) same level of difficulty, and (c) similar grammatical construct (e.g. either past or present tense).

Daily interaction with students is an excellent source of good quality distracters. Experienced teachers know the common mistakes that students are likely to make and the sources of their confusion. They can identify common deficiencies in students' knowledge and faults in their reasoning process. Usually there are recognizable and recurrent patterns of students' mistakes, confusions, and deficiencies. Experienced and astute teachers also know the important 'must know' situations. All these factors can be utilized to construct good quality distracters.

Examples of MCQ With Hierarchical Cognitive Objectives

From the previous sections we have learned that the assessment of knowledge acquisition and comprehension is generally over-represented in MCQ based examinations. Careful incorporation of charts, diagrams, photographs, tables, and other visual materials enhances variety but does not necessarily equate to assessment of higher order cognitive abilities. It may appear counterintuitive, but the difficulty of a question does not correlate consistently with testing of higher order cognitive abilities. For example, a MCQ may be very difficult but still tests knowledge recall. Likewise, a MCQ may not be that difficult but yet can adequately test higher order cognitive abilities.

In the following paragraphs, our tasks are to examine ways of constructing MCQ for various levels in the cognitive domains including higher orders. Readers are urged to make frequent reference to two earlier chapters (a) Classification of Educational Objectives (Chapter Eight) and (b) Writing Educational Objectives (Chapter Nine) to correlate between educational objectives and construction of MCQ.

This patient scenario is for Question One to Question Five:

JK is an extremely premature baby with broncho-pulmonary dysplasia (BPD). She is on mechanical ventilator and receiving oral diuretics (chlorthiazide and spironolactone) therapy for her problem. You are about to start Dexamethasone for BPD.

Question one

Cognitive level: Knowledge
Question objective: Recognize the side effects of Dexamethasone in premature babies.
Test question: Which of the following is NOT a recognized side effect of Dexamethasone therapy?

A. Weight loss
B. Hypertension
C. Infection
D. Hypoglycemia
E. Rickets
(Answer D)

Note: Students' task is limited to knowing and recognizing the side effects of Dexamethasone. There is little or no comprehension necessary to answer the question.

Question two

Cognitive level: Comprehension
Question objective: Interpret the acid-base imbalances.
Test question: JK was mechanically ventilated. The analysis of arterial blood gas and electrolytes revealed the following parameters:

pH	7.36	Sodium	132 mmol/L
PCO_2	64 mm of Hg	Potassium	4.6 mmol/L
PO_2	61 mm of Hg	Chloride	101 mmol/L
HCO_3	32 mmol/L		
Base excess	+ 11 mmol/L		

Which of the following best describe JK's acid-base status?

A. Acute respiratory alkalosis, no metabolic compensation
B. Acute metabolic alkalosis
C. Normal acid-base status
D. Chronic respiratory acidosis, with metabolic compensation
E. Chronic metabolic alkalosis
(Answer: D)

Note: Students are required to understand (i.e. comprehend) the acid-base imbalance. Simple knowledge recall is insufficient to answer the question. But the question falls short of getting the students to correlate laboratory findings with patient's clinical status—a higher level characteristic of 'analysis'.

Question three

Cognitive level: Analysis
Question objective: Analysis of acid-base status and correlation with patient's clinical status.
Test question: Which of the following clinical scenarios is the most likely explanation of JK's acid-base status?

A. Chronic hypo-ventilation
B. Acute onset of pneumonia
C. Acute broncho-spasm
D. Renal insufficiency
E. Chronic over ventilation
(Answer A)

Note: This question requires interpretation of the laboratory values and correlation with the clinical status. This is a step forward from the previous question.

Question four

Cognitive Level: Application
Question objective: Calculate appropriate correction of electrolyte imbalance.

Test question: Several days later, JK's serum electrolyte shows the following pattern

Sodium   118 mmol/L
Potassium   5.7 mmol/L
Chloride   83 mmol/L

You have decided to correct the sodium imbalance. Your target level of sodium after the correction is 130 mmol/L. JK's current weight is one kilogram. How much sodium (in mmol) JK will be needed to bring up her sodium to the desired level?

A. 12
B. 7.2
C. 5.9
D. 3.6
E. None of the above
(Answer: B)

Note: This question requires application of a common formula for the correction of sodium deficit to the patient's problem. In situations that require computation 'None of the above' as a final option makes the questions more discriminatory as the unsure student does not focus on a set of answers that contain an answer. (Although the application level is lower than analysis it is placed here for the smooth flow of the patient scenario).

Cognitive Level: Synthesis
Synthesis level requires proposition and development of something new such as a patient's management or diagnostic work-up plan. As such, the synthesis level is better assessed with open-ended questions rather than restrictive response questions such as MCQ.

Question five

Cognitive Level: Evaluation
Question objective: Compare and choose a correct management approach from a variety of plausible alternatives.

Test question: Based on JK's current electrolyte imbalance, you have ordered some investigations. Pending the results of these tests, what immediate management option is MOST suitable in this situation?

A. Discontinuation of both chlorthiazide and spironolactone and careful observation over the next 24 hours
B. Slow correction (over 24 hours) of serum sodium, correction of potassium by administering IV lasix
C. Slow correction (over 24 hours) of serum sodium, discontinuation of both chlorthiazide and spironolactone
D. Slow correction (over 24 hours) of serum sodium and discontinuation of chlorthiazide
E. Rapid correction (over 6 hours) of serum sodium and discontinuation of both chlorthiazide and spironolactone
(Answer: C)

Note: The choices that are presented here are all plausible. The students have to judge and choose the best modality over the others.

Mere comparison without utilization of judgement does not constitute an evaluation level question. Consider the following example:

Test question: You have decided to compare between inhaled steroid and systemic steroid for the management of BPD in premature babies. Which of the following types of article is likely to provide the best evidence for your question?

A. A published guideline
B. A systematic review
C. A randomized control trial
D. A case control study
E. Opinion from an expert panel
(Answer C)

In this example, although it requires comparison between the choices, the question can be easily answered by simple memory recall. There is no judgement involved in this case. This is an example of a pseudo-evaluation level question and is discouraged.

In medical education, it is highly recommended that *MCQ integrate concepts from basic science and clinical science*. Recently, National Board of Medical Examiners reiterated the importance of using clinical scenarios in both Step I (former basic science) and Step II (former clinical science) examinations. In the following examples, it is readily evident how clinical vignettes are used in writing good quality MCQ that tests many higher order cognitive abilities that are highlighted above.

Good MCQ

A middle-aged male complains of difficulty climbing the stairs. He describes weakness without pain in his right lower limb. He is able to place his right leg on each step without experiencing any problem, but has difficulty climbing the step, and must grasp the hand-rail to pull himself up. Climbing the next step with his left leg occurs normally. You also notice that his gait on a flat surface appears nearly normal; there is no weakness in extending the right knee against a considerable load. You suspect damage and/or malfunction in the

  A. Obturator nerve
  B. Tibial nerve
  C. Superior gluteal nerve
  D. Femoral nerve
  E. Inferior gluteal nerve (correct option)

Poor MCQ

A glycolytic conversion of glucose to lactate:

  A. Generates *net* gain of two NADH's for each glucose consumed
  B. Requires the direct participation of molecular oxygen
  C. Cannot take place in the cells lacking mitochondria
  D. Is stimulated by a high intracellular concentration of fructose- 2,6- bis-phosphate (correct option)
  E. Involves a *single* dehydrogenase

In most cases of sensorineural (inner ear damage) hearing loss:

A. Hearing improves with time
B. Surgery can correct the loss
C. Removal of the cochlea is recommended
D. High-frequency hearing is lost before low-frequency hearing
E. Amplifying incoming sounds will correct all perceptual problem (correct option)

From: Jozefowicz RF, Koeppen BM, Case S, Galbraith R, Swanson D, Glew RH. The Quality of In-house Examinations. *Academic Medicine*. 2002. 77(2) 156–61. Used with permission.

Further Improvements in MCQ

Although MCQ offer objectivity and relatively wider domain sampling that is attractive for student assessment, their value is somewhat limited as they are considered as restricted option questions. Students are required to choose a particular item from a range of given selections. To alleviate the problem an alternate form of assessment method is necessary where virtually all the possibilities are given as options. This format is known as Extended Matching Item (EMI). In a way, EMI are practical alternatives to open-response questions while maintaining the objectivity and consistency (Case and Swanson, 1993).

EMI test the application of knowledge and allow easy incorporation of clinical vignette into basic science context. They also allow greater discriminatory power over limited choice MCQ as the responses are widely distributed (Case and Swanson, 1994).

Let us consider the following example.
Content focus: Respiratory distress in newborn
Instruction: For each of the patient scenario below choose the most likely diagnosis.

Question 1: A new born baby is found to have grunting and tachypnea immediately after birth. The baby was born by normal vaginal delivery after 34 weeks of gestational age. The mother had infrequent follow-up and suffered from uncontrollable diabetes during pregnancy. The baby's chest x-ray shows ground-glass appearance. His total white count is 18,000/ml, immature to total neutrophil ratio is 0.04.

Question 2: A four-hour old baby developed grunting and tachypnea. He was born by caesarian section after 39 weeks of gestational age. His chest x-ray shows fluid in horizontal fissure in the right lung. His white count is 17,000/ml, immature to total neutrophil ratio is 0.08.

Options:

A. Pneumothorax
B. Pleural effusion
C. Tracheomalacia
D. Pneumonia
E. Hyaline membrane disease
F. Transient tachypnea of newborn
G. Septicemia
H. Anemia
I. Polycythemia
J. Hypoglycemia
K. Hypothermia
L. Ventricular-septal defect
M. Meconium aspiration syndrome
N. Coarctation of aorta
O. Broncho-pulmonary dysplasia
P. Tracheo-esophageal fistula

Note that the options include essentially all plausible causes of respiratory distress in newborn. The greater range of options allows more discrimination than the limited choice MCQ (Case and Swanson, 1993 & 1994).

Evaluating MCQ

The worthiness of any assessment method includes the ability to judge whether a particular student has achieved a minimum competency and to differentiate between better students from mediocre ones. A test item that is too easy for anyone to answer or a test item that is too difficult that nobody can answer is not helpful in achieving the above two goals. A test item should be difficult enough to assess competency level and be of such quality that most of the knowledgeable students would be able to answer the questions whereas the mediocre students would not. Difficulty and discriminatory indices are two objective ways of demonstrating the concept and widely used in the evaluation of MCQ.

Difficulty index: This refers to how difficult (or easy) the test item is to answer. This is the proportion between the number of students who answered the item correctly and the total number of students taking the examination and expressed as a fractional number or percentage. For example, a difficulty index of 55% refers to the fact that 55% of the students who sat for the examination were able to answer the question correctly. Note that the higher the number, the *easier* it is to answer. An ideal difficulty index is 50–60%, but 30–70% is acceptable in most situations (Guilbert, 1981).

Discrimination index: This determines how well a test item differentiates between knowledgeable and mediocre students. The discrimination index is calculated by following the steps below

- Step 1: Rank all the students in order according to their performance in the test.
- Step 2: Divide the group more or less equally in four quarters. The lowest quartile (25%) is the low performing group and the highest quartile (25%) is the high performing group.
- Step 3: Calculate the discrimination index using the following formula

$$\text{Discrimination Index} = 2\text{x}\frac{H - L}{N} \tag{1}$$

H = number of correct answers in High Group
L = number of correct answers in Low Group
N = combined number of students in both groups

The discrimination index can range from -1 to +1. The higher the index the more likely the question will differentiate between 'high' and 'low' students for that given group. Discrimination index of .35 or above is considered excellent, index between 0.25–0.35 is acceptable, whereas any question with index of < 0.25 needs revision (Guilbert, 1981).

The evaluation process is further enhanced by systemic representation of essential information of each test item. A 3X5 card is an easy way of cataloging such data. In the following example, A–E refers to the options in the question and corresponding numbers are percentage of answers. Besides providing a graphic and objective overview of each of the question, this card also points to the most and the least useful options. In this example, options A and B have very little discriminatory power as both 'High' and 'Low' students choose these options equally. These options need revision.

Target Student: Final Year			Subject: Pediatrics/Neonatology		
Objective: Analysis of acid base imbalances in newborn and identification of the clinical status					
Difficulty Index: 76 Discriminatory Index: 0.30			Correct answer: D		
Answers in High Group	A: 3%	B: 5%	C: 2%	D: 88%	E: 2%
Answers in Low Group	A: 4%	B: 6%	C: 10%	D: 65%	E: 15%

Currently, there are many commercial software programs available that provide a comprehensive profile of test items.

In summary, the key points that we have learned in this chapter are

- MCQ test knowledge (cognition) but are inefficient in assessing attitudes and skills
- MCQ can assess higher order cognitive functions
- MCQ are favored as they test large content area quickly with a high degree of reliability and consistency
- Incorporation of clinical vignette and integration of basic and clinical science knowledge are recommended in MCQ
- In EMI the number of options are much higher and include all plausible ones
- EMI offer greater discrimination than limited choice MCQ
- Difficulty and discriminatory indices are used to determine the effectiveness of MCQ and EMI

Formal Training Improves Question Quality

A group of researchers assessed the quality of in-house multiple choice questions from three US medical schools. They have used blind assessment and predetermined criteria in a five point Likert's scale (Score 1= tested recall only and was technically flawed; score 5= used a laboratory or clinical vignette, required reasoning to answer, and free of technical flaws). Questions written by examiners without formal training in test writing had a mean score of 2.03; whereas questions written by examiners with formal training in test writing had a mean score of 4.24. The authors drew the valid conclusion that the quality of in-house examination can be significantly improved by providing question writers with formal training.

Jozefowicz RF, *et al*. The Quality of In-house Examinations. *Academic Medicine*. 2002. 77(2) 156–61.

References and Further Readings

1. Case SM, and Swanson DB. Extended Matching Items: A Practical Alternative to Free-Response Questions. *Teaching and Learning in Medicine*. 1993. 5(2): 107–115.
2. Case SM, Swanson DB, and Ripkey DR. Comparison of Items in Five-option and Extended Matching Format for Assessment of Diagnostic Skills. *Academic Medicine*. 1994. 69 (Supplement): S1–S3.
3. Case SM, Swanson DB, and Becker D. Verbosity, Window Dressing, and Red Herrings: Do They Make a Better Test Item? *Academic Medicine*. 1996. 71(10 Suppl): S 28–30.
4. Case SM, and Swanson DB. *Constructing Written Test Questions for the Basic and Clinical Sciences*. Third Edition. National Board of Medical Examiners. Philadelphia, PA. 1998. Web address: http://www.nbme.org/nbme/itemwriting.htm Accessed May

02. (An excellent and comprehensive 'how to' guide for test item writings)

5. Jozefowicz RF, Koeppen BM, Case S, Galbraith R, Swanson D, and Glew RH. The Quality of In-house Examinations. *Academic Medicine*. 2002. 77(2) 156–61.

6. Guilbert J-J. *Educational Handbook for Health Personnel*. 1981. Revised Edition. WHO Offset Publication No 35. World Health Organization, Geneva.

7. Schultheis NM. Writing Cognitive Educational Objectives and Multiple Choice Test Questions. *The American Journal of Health-System Pharmacists*. 1998 (55): 2397–401.

32 Essay Questions and Variations

For many years, essay questions, especially the longer version, used to be the main assessment tool in medical schools. It is still in use in many parts of the world. Concerns about their lack of objective scoring prompted medical schools either to gradually phase them out or to receive less weightage during assessment. There are also modified and structured essay questions more suitable for summative assessment.

In this chapter, our tasks are to

- Identify the features of different types of essay question
- Determine their proper applications and utilizations
- Construct and critically review examples of various types of essay question

After reading the chapter, we should be able to compose different types of essay question suitable for student assessment.

Road Map to Student Assessment

    What does it assess?
    Knowledge   Attitude   Skill

    The level of knowledge
    Knows   **Knows how**   Shows how   Does

    Utility as summative assessment
    Yes   No

    Validity (content)
    High   **Medium**   Low

    Reliability
    High   **Medium**   Low

Advantages

The major advantage of an essay question is its potential ability to assess higher level cognitive functions. This is an open form of question that can encourage students into critical thinking; they are compelled to analyze underlying facts, synthesize and propose new ideas, and provide reasons for the preferred choice.

An essay question also assesses the students' ability to collate and organize information and ideas. Students are required to present their ideas in a succinct and logical way that would make sense to others. For the examiners, the advantage is that it is relatively easy to construct.

Advantages of Essay Question

- Good for assessment of higher order cognitive functions
- Promotion of critical thinking
- Presentation of loose ideas in an organized and logical manner
- Ease of construction

Challenges and Limitations

However, essay type question has several disadvantages and challenges, the most important of which is relative lack of reliability and consistency in scoring. Significant inter-rater as well as intra-rater variabilities are common during marking of essay questions. In addition, if the scope of the question is not broad enough, essay questions tend to test only a limited amount of knowledge from the content and thereby compromise the content validity. These problems are more pronounced with longer type of essay questions and can be remedied, but not completely eliminated, by creating several shorter form of questions and with careful attention to creation of model answers.

Limitations of Essay Question

- Relative lack of reliability and consistency
- Intra-rater and inter-rater variability in scoring
- Limited content coverage
- Limited content validity

Common misuse of essay type questions includes testing for knowledge recall; ignoring fuller capabilities of these questions. Frequent use of 'restricted response words' such as *'what'*, *'list'*, *'when'* accentuates the problem. For example, 'What are the side-effects of digoxin?' is a restricted response question that tests knowledge recall. Words with higher cognitive value, such as *'compare and contrast'*, *'provide argument for'*, are preferred alternatives, as they improve question quality significantly.

Students' acceptance of essay questions improves if they are made familiar with this assessment method and the course pre-empts them about the expected questions and their answer forms. Students may not know the meaning of many key operative terms (e.g. propose, validate, evaluate, compare) in the questions or interpret them differently. The problem can be alleviated by using similar question styles with key operative terms during the course.

Classroom discussion should also reflect the expected questions asked during examination.

Basic Categories of Essay Questions

Essay questions fall into two broad categories depending upon the format and scope of the answer: (a) extended response and (b) restricted response.

Extended response questions allow students considerable freedom and latitude to answer. The expected answers are non-restrictive; divergent viewpoints are generally expected and encouraged. As such, extended response questions are more suitable for assessment of attributes such as proposition, evaluation, and synthesis.

> Example: You are a committee member in charge of implementing 'Healthy Life-Style Campaign' in the community. As a health care provider, *propose* a plan of actions to the committee to reduce cardiovascular morbidity and mortality in the community.

Restricted response questions limit the choice of responses and set the boundary for the answer. Expected answers are somewhat narrower in their scope and more convergent than the extended response questions. As there are certain limitations imposed on the students in answering the questions, restricted response questions are less efficacious for assessing higher order cognitive functions compared to extended response questions.

> Example: Describe the pharmacological management of a child with acute asthma that you have seen in the out-patient clinic. Argue in favor of your choice of the medications.

Generally speaking, the longer form of essay question allows assessment of higher cognitive functions, but lacks reliability and consistency in scoring. With shorter forms of essay question, reliability and consistency can be improved but these come with a compromise—the question becomes less efficient in assessing higher cognitive functions.

In medical education, modified forms of essay questions are in use as both summative and formative assessment instruments. Short answer question (SAQ) and modified essay question (MEQ) are examples of two such formats. Both SAQ and MEQ are semi-structured objective assessment tools with better reliability and objectivity than the long essay question format. Structurally they are more akin to restricted response questions and more convenient for assessing specific content areas such as history taking, physical examination findings, interpretation of laboratory and radiological data, and patient management plan.

Short Answer Questions (SAQ)

SAQ have several advantages that make them attractive for both the examiners and the students. SAQ can be used to cover broader content areas by asking several discrete and important questions about the topic and thereby improving content validity. The scoring is easier and better as the answers are specific and short. The reliability is improved with standard predetermined answers for each question set by the examiners.

SAQ are generally constructed around a theme or patient scenario followed by several focused questions. These questions may include key features, comparisons, mechanism of actions, side effects etc. Each question bears separate mark that is clearly indicated in the question paper. The total duration of time for answering the question is usually comparable or shorter than long essay questions.

Example
Question focus: Neonates and children with meningitis.

Question 1: What are the clinical features of neonatal meningitis?

Question 2: What are the features in the cerebro-spinal fluid that separate bacterial meningitis from viral meningitis?

Question 3: What are the complications of bacterial meningitis in children?

Modified Essay Questions (MEQ)

A slight variation to the short answer question is the modified essay question. MEQ are constructed around a specific theme or a patient scenario that is presented in the beginning. The questions are revealed to the students in a sequential manner and more information about the case is revealed to the students in steps. The sequence of information presented resembles real-life, thus bringing in realism and improving face validity. Just like real-life cases, students may not revert back to earlier segments once the answer is already completed. With careful attention, MEQ can be designed to test problem solving and decision making ability of students.

Two other specific features of MEQ deserve special attention. First, the stem of later questions may provide clues for answers to earlier questions especially when a patient's scenario is presented. Second, as the questions are connected to each other, there is a chance that the students will be penalized repeatedly for the same error.

Example of MEQ:
(Sample model answers are presented)
Instruction: This is a common clinical scenario in neonates. Answer the questions as they appear. There may be more answers than has been listed in the questions. If so, choose more important responses first. Just like clinical cases, information will be provided to you sequentially and you may not revert back to earlier sections.
You have TWENTY MINUTES to complete TWENTY QUESTIONS.

All answers carry equal number of marks. Keep a steady pace so that you can answer ALL the questions.

Questions 1–5

Tara is a new born baby. She was born by caesarian section at 36 weeks of gestational age because of persistent tachycardia noted in a cardio-tocogram. She developed respiratory distress immediately after delivery. Name five common causes of respiratory distress that can give rise to Tara's problem.

(Model answers: Transient tachypnoea of newborn, pneumonia and sepsis, peumothorax, meconium aspiration syndrome, hyaline membrane disease, hypothermia, anemia, congenital cyanotic heart diseases).

Questions 6–7

Her vitals are HR 134/min, RR 72/minute, and temperature 35.4 C. Which of these values are considered abnormal for a neonate?

(Model answers: Respiratory rate and temperature)

Questions 8–11

List four signs of respiratory distress in newborn.

(Model answers: Tachypnoea, flaring of ala nasae, grunting, and retractions.)

Questions 12–15

List four historical information about Tara's mother during her pregnancy and labor that you need to help you narrow down the diagnostic possibilities.

(Model answers: Diabetes, history of infections, prolonged rupture of membrane, UTI, Apgar scores, amniotic fluid characteristics)

Questions 17–18

Tara's mother did not have any major illness throughout the pregnancy. Routine antenatal ultrasounds were normal. She did not have any history of leaking amniotic fluid. Although she had fever, dysuria, and increased frequency of urine for the last few days. Tara's Apgar scores were six and eight at one and five minutes of life. You have decided to treat Tara for possible infection. What are

the features in full blood count that suggest infection in the newborn?
(Model answers: High or very low total white cell counts, elevated immature to mature neutrophil ratios)

Questions 19–20
What are the antibiotics that can be used as an initial therapy for presumptive sepsis in Tara?
(Model answers: Ampicillin and Gentamicin.)
END OF CASE

Before utilizing essay type question for student assessment, we need to make sure this is the correct type of instrument for that specific purpose and there is no better alternative for that. Also, we need to decide the better essay question format for the purpose—a long essay question or several shorter alternatives. Whatever the format of the questions, determination of model answers and scoring methods is imperative to improve consistency and reliability in scoring.

In summary, the important points that we learned are

- Well-written essay questions are good for assessment of higher order cognitive functions such as proposition, synthesis, and evaluation
- The main concerns are relatively low content coverage and relative lack of reliability and consistency in scoring
- Several short questions provide better content coverage and make the scoring easier and more consistent
- Pre-determination of answers and grading criteria is essential before using essay questions as summative assessment tools

References and Further Readings

1. Cantillon P. Mastering Exam Technique. *British Medical Journal.* The web address: http://www.studentbmj.com/back_issues /1000/education/363.html; accessed July 02.

2. Ebel RL. *Essential of Educational Measurements*. 1979. Prentice-Hall Incorporated. Englewood Cliff. NJ. USA.

33 Oral Examinations

Oral examination format should continue only if there are efforts by the Examining Board to "review, improve, and educate itself ...striving always for greater objectivity and ...validity"

Pope WDB

The oral examination has a long tradition in medical education as a summative assessment instrument. It is still used by many schools and professional certifying bodies while many others have dropped it or modified the traditional form extensively. Others use oral examination as a form of formative assessment to aid in learning.

In this chapter, our tasks are to

- Discuss the advantages and shortcomings of oral examination
- Identify situations where oral examinations are appropriate
- Determine some ways to improve the validity and reliability of this form of examination

Road Map to Student Assessment

What does it assess?

Knowledge	Attitude	Skill

The level of knowledge

Knows	Knows how	Shows how	Does

Utility as summative assessment

Questionable

Validity

High	Medium	Low

Reliability

High	Medium	Low

Advantages

The oral examination provides several advantages that are not readily available with other forms of examination. One of these advantages that has a very high utility in medical education is the assessment of 'clinical competence.' Assessment of clinical competence requires determination of a student's strengths in several domains such as clinical reasoning and problem solving skills, ability to prioritize and evaluate competing management options, and defending his own decisions. The oral examination, if administered by a trained examiner, provides valuable insights into the student's ability in these relatively abstract domains. Many other forms of student assessment methods may not address these issues sufficiently.

The oral examination also allows face to face interactions between the examiners and examinee allowing on the spot assessment of students' strengths and weaknesses in a particular area. It also provides opportunity for immediate feedback.

The oral examination also allows limited assessment of communication skills, linguistic ability and other aspects of interpersonal relationship, although there are more valid and reliable instruments available for these purposes.

Advantages of Oral Examination

- Allows assessment of
    - Reasoning and deductive processes
    - Problem solving
    - Capacity to defend decisions
    - Evaluation of competing choices
    - Ability to prioritize
- Face to face interaction
- Provides flexibility to concentrate on one content area
- Explores students' viewpoints

Practice of these features during examinations *requires a high level of training and motivation of the examiners.*

Oral examination as a form of *formative assessment* has substantial usefulness in medical education. Teachers find oral examination attractive as this allows insight into the students' reasoning and decision-making processes and opportunity for feedback.

Limitations

The first and foremost objection to using oral examination as a summative assessment method is the lack of reliability and consistency in scoring. The unreliability or inconsistency in the examination potentially can originate from various sources including examiners, examinee, and the format. The oral examination is prone to intra-rater and inter-rater variability. For example, there is significant 'halo effect' where an examiner's overall judgment of the candidate's competency is seriously flawed by external appearance or other inconsequential attributes of the examinee. Lack of reliability also results from variations in question determination or case selection during the examination.

There is a poor correlation between the oral examination and other forms of examination that are commonly practiced in medical education. One of the possible explanations is that oral examination tends to assess a *different* aspect of competency in students than the other forms of examination—a point that is perceived favorably by many. The content coverage in the oral examination also tends to be limited, thereby compromising the content validity. Examiners have insufficient time to assess the students' breadth of knowledge.

Concerns for Oral Examinations

- Lack of standardization and reproducibility
- Limited coverage of content area
- Lack of transparency
- Prone to biases such as external appearances of the students
- Fear of manipulation and favoritism
- Lack of record keeping of the examination process
- High manpower resource utilization
- Undue anxiety among the students

The above deficiencies are more pronounced in unstructured oral examination. Both the validity and reliability can be improved with examiners' education, standardization, and instilling structure to the examination process.

Improving the Validity and Reliability of Oral Examinations

Institutes and organizations that have successfully practiced oral examination as a summative assessment instrument are able to do so because of a high degree of institutional commitment to improve the standard of student assessment and continuous appraisal of the examination process. Both the examiners and examinee need to be aware of, in addition to fundamental aspects of assessment process, the purpose of oral examination, specific attributes that the examination intends to test, and its shortcomings.

The structure of the oral examination can be modified to improve validity and reliability thereby reducing variability of examinations. The issue of lack of reliability and objectivity is addressed by creation of a set of standardized questions with answer. The questions are posed to the examinee in a random manner. Furthermore, uniform grading criteria need to be developed *a priori* to determine the accepted and unaccepted answers. The entire process usually requires several rounds of discussion among the examiners and pilot testing in simulated situations.

The issue of transparency and record keeping is addressed by having clear instructions to the examinee regarding what they are expected to face in the examination and how they would be judged. Ideally a third examiner is employed to record the verbal interchange (both questions and answers) between the examiners and examinee. Record keeping is strongly encouraged if the oral examination is to be used as a certifying examination.

Content validity of oral examination is improved with a longer examination format and broader domain sampling. The longer examination format brings stability in the examination process and makes it less variable.

To illustrate the level of commitment needed let us consider the Canadian Anesthesia Society's certification examination that employs oral examination for the purpose (Kearney, 02). The oral examination is supplemented by written examination. The oral examination consists of two sessions. In each session, three examiners ask the candidate five standardized questions over one hour. Two examiners ask the questions and third examiner records the candidate's responses. All three examiners score the candidate on an anchored global scale in a blinded manner. The second session is similar to the first session but with a different set of examiners (Kearney, 02). Note—the length of the examination is two hours, usage of specific number of standardized question, use of predetermined rating scale, and blinded scoring. Also, as the third examiner records the responses it addresses the issue of record keeping and transparency. Analysis of this examination format points to several important aspects that we have discussed earlier. It also illustrates the high degree of training that is needed to ensure the required degree of consistency, objectivity and validity.

Format of Oral Examination to Improve Validity and Reliability

- Consensus on the definitions of operative terms;
  e.g. problem solving, critical reasoning
- Standard predetermined questions
- Predetermined model answers
- Pre-agreed rating scale
- Blind independent scoring
- Longer examination

Oral examination has an unquestionable beneficial role of assessing critical analysis, problem solving, and reasoning process. As these attributes are essential elements of clinical competence, oral examinations can be especially helpful in medical education. But to use it as a form of effective and unbiased summative assessment requires considerable institutional and individual commitment to train examiners in this assessment form.

In summary, the key points that we have learned are

- Oral examination is useful to assess critical reasoning and problem solving
- Unstructured oral examinations seriously lack the desired level of validity and reliability as a summative assessment tool
- Oral examination is valuable for formative assessment
- Validity and reliability of the oral examination can be improved through faculty education and by instilling proper structure

References and Further Readings

1. Kearney RA, Puchalski SA, Homer YH, and Yang. The Inter-Rater and Intra-Rater Reliability of a New Canadian Oral Examination Format in Anesthesia is Fair to Good. *Canadian Journal of Anesthesia*. 2002. 49(3): 232–36.
2. Muzzin LJ, and Hart I. Oral Examination. In: Neufeld VR, Norman GR (eds). *Assessing Clinical Competence*. Springer Publishing Company. New York. USA. 1985. 71–93.
3. Pope WDB. Anesthesia Oral Examination (editorial). *Canadian Journal of Anesthesia*. 1993. 40: 907–10.

34 Standardized Patient

Standardized patient or SP is one of the most significant innovations in medical education. Dr. Howard Barrows first used the term 'programmed patient' to describe lay persons who are trained to simulate a patient. The original role of SP was as a convenient and effective teaching tool to demonstrate physical findings in clinical settings. Over the last two decades its uses have broadened considerably and SP has now become an integral part of both *teaching* and *assessment*.

In this chapter, our tasks are to

- Identify the strengths and advantages of standardized patient
- Determine the implementation considerations of standardized patient program
- Identify situations where standardized patient is an appropriate assessment instrument

After completing the chapter and with help of a few other additional resources that are listed in the reference section, you should be able to develop 'Standardized Patient Blueprint' and effectively act as a member of 'Standardized Patient Development Team.'

Road Map to Student Assessment

What does it assess?
Knowledge   Attitude   **Skill**

The level of application
Knows   **Knows how**   **Shows how**   Does

Utility as summative assessment
Yes   No

Validity (Construct)
High   Medium   Low

Reliability
High   **Medium**   Low

The standardized patients are people, either real patients or laypersons, who have been carefully *coached and trained to portray a patient in a standardized manner*. Such portrayal is varied from simulating the entire patient to isolated attributes such as historical and physical findings, body language, emotion, and personality characteristics. A similar term 'simulated patient' is often used as well. Barrows proposed separate definitions to demarcate simulated patient and standardized patient. His suggested definition of simulated patient is a 'normal person who has been carefully coached to accurately portray a specific patient when given the history and physical findings.' He recommended reserving the term standardized patient 'as a broader umbrella for both simulated patients and actual patients who have been carefully coached to present their own illnesses in a standardized, unvarying way.' (Barrows, 93). We will follow Barrows' definition and use the term SP patient to indicate both simulated patient and actual patients who are coached and standardized.

Standardized patients come from all walks of life. Some of them are professional or amateur actors; others are lay persons, while a few of them are actual patients. Some of the medical schools have used medical students successfully as standardized patients. Generally, a selected number of standardized patients receive additional training to assess the clinical skills of the students and provide constructive feedback during the encounters.

Why Do We Need Standardized Patients?

Assessment of clinical competence in the student is unique in medicine. Assessment of clinical competence is recognized as the most valid representation of the students' ability to master medicine as this closely simulates what he is expected to do in real life. Accordingly, the student assessment system should incorporate some assessment techniques to test students' ability in this particular area. The paper and pencil based assessment techniques fall significantly short of assessing clinical competence. Mostly they either test knowledge only or do not realistically portray clinical encounters. Student assessment methods that involve patients are more valid for assessment of clinical competence.

However, involvement of patients in the student assessment poses a new challenge. Each patient is unique. The disease manifestations, physical and psychological profiles, and expectations from the caregiver are a few of the many attributes that are essentially unique to individual patient. From an assessment viewpoint, all these personal attributes and idiosyncrasies are 'confounding variables' that make the assessment system less consistent, hence less reliable. Standardization of patients counteracts the problem by creating more uniformity and less variability in terms of disease characterizations and portrayal. Moreover, standardization also involves uniform and predetermined grading criteria.

In short, the 'patient' component in the standardized patient improves the validity of assessment of clinical competence whereas 'standardization' enhances the reliability and consistency.

Uses

In clinical medicine, SP is effectively used to portray a full range of clinical encounters including history taking, performing physical examinations, decision making exercises, and counseling. During history taking, SP can demonstrate required body language, personality traits and a wide range of emotional status to add realism during the interview. A trained SP can convincingly portray an astonishing range of physical examination findings (Barrows, 99). The possibility includes relatively simple findings such as neck rigidity, various gait abnormalities, acute abdomen etc. With little imagination and ingenuity, other seemingly impossible findings such as hypertension, jaundice, or dilated pupils can be demonstrated with confidence.

Besides demonstrating clinical examination findings, the SP can be effective tools for teachers to get insight about students' decision making and reasoning skills. SP can be of significant value to teach and practice a wide range of counseling and communication skills.

The use of SP in student assessment is relatively new. The SP can be used in conjunction with Objective Structured Clinical Examination (OSCE) where the students are required to act on a specific problem like eliciting pertinent history of a diabetic patient or examination of lower limb. The SP can also be used as a stand alone case during longer examinations where the students are required to obtain a comprehensive history, perform physical examination, devise a management plan, and counsel the patients.

Advantages

Properly trained SP provides many advantages for both clinical teachers and medical students during teaching and assessment.

- *Validity*
  SP is a highly valid tool for student assessment. During a clinical examination SP can measure what a clinical examination is supposed to measure—history taking, clinical skills, reasoning and decision making skills, and counseling.
- *Reliability*
  The portrayal of patient problems in SP is standardized. Unlike real patients, standardized patients are trained to main-

tain high degree of consistency from one encounter to another.

- *Objectivity*

  As the patient problems are standardized and uniform, it is much easier for independent examiners to agree on the grading.

- *Availability*

  A common concern among clinical teachers is the lack of availability of patients to demonstrate particular condition in time of need. A pool of SP allows clinical teachers to choose easily from a wide variety of conditions.

- *Patient safety and privacy*

  There is increasing concern about exposing real patients to repeated examinations. Use of SP ensures that patients do not experience unnecessary and often-prolonged examination by the novice.

- *Acute and difficult cases*

  SP can effectively portray emergency situations and difficult cases that are not commonly encountered by medical students yet vital for them to know. Examples of such cases include approach to unconscious patient, upper airway obstructions, etc.

- *Feedback*

  A trained SP can provide immediate feedback to the medical students after the encounter.

Strengths of Standardized Patient

- Probably the most valid tool for assessment of clinical skills
- Better reliability and objectivity than real patients
- Easy availability
- Protection of patient privacy and safety
- Immediate feedback

Implementation Considerations

There are several important implementation considerations for using standardized patient. The preparation time is longer as it includes script writing, training of the standardized patient, and pilot testing. It may take several sessions for someone to become familiar with the case and realistically portray the findings in a consistent manner.

The budgetary need to run a successful SP program is a valid concern. Encouragingly such monetary requirement is not high. For example, hourly remuneration for standardized patients in the US is about US $12–16. In Singapore, a few institutions have used standardized patients for teaching purposes. They were paid approximately S$15 per hour.

Often times, concerns are raised about the SP's ability to demonstrate required range of physical findings. As discussed earlier, this is not a limiting factor and the range of medical conditions that can be successfully portrayed by the standardized patient is far more numerous than most of us imagine. Furthermore, patients with fixed medical problems or findings (e.g. cardiac murmur, facial nerve palsy) can be trained to become standardized patients as well.

Beyond these logistic issues, another important consideration is that SP is clinical encounter specific. As such, SP is not efficient enough to assess a large body of knowledge. The SP is generally supplemented with alternate assessment instruments that are more efficient in testing larger body of knowledge.

The development of standardized patient is a team effort. Typically such a team consists of a scriptwriter (physician), medical education specialist, and a standardized patient trainer. Physicians provide the scripts that can be based on real patients with necessary modifications.

Implementation Considerations

- Professional expertise and experience
- Preparation time
- Budgetary requirement
- Limited domain sampling

In Appendix B, there is a Standardized Patient Blue Print that can be used as a prototype for the development of other cases.

In summary, the important points that we have learned are

- Standardized patient is a valid and reliable way of assessment of clinical competence
- Standardized patient provides many advantages over traditional paper and pencil based test in clinical competence assessment
- Wide range of acute and chronic, physical and psychological characteristics can be accurately portrayed
- Standardized patient development team is recommended for the successful implementation of standardized patient program

References and Further Readings

1. Barrows HS. An Overview of the Uses of Standardized Patients for Teaching and Evaluating Clinical Skills. *Academic Medicine.* 1993. 68 (9): 443–53.
2. Barrows HS. *Training Standardized Patients to Have Physical Findings.* 1999. Southern Illinois University. Springfield, IL. USA.
3. King AM, Perkowski-Rogers LC, and Pohl HS. Planning Standardized Patient Programs: Case Development, Patient Training, and Costs. *Teaching and Learning in Medicine.* 1994. 6(1): 6–14.

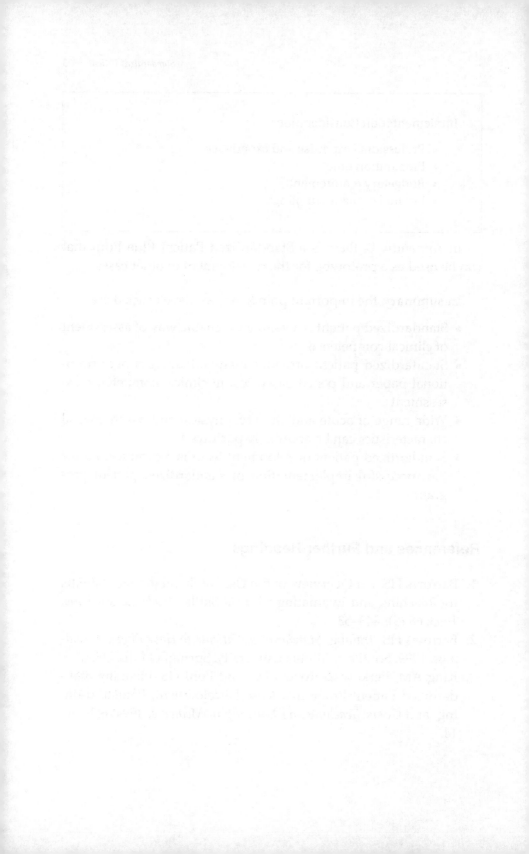

35 Portfolio

Portfolio assessment in medical education is a relatively new concept. There is considerable interest in portfolio as this is widely believed to support student-centered and self-directed learning and assessment. Portfolio is useful both as a *learning and assessment tool*. We will discuss portfolio from both perspectives and demonstrate its value as a process as well as an outcome.

In this chapter, our tasks are to

- Discuss the definition, scopes, and purposes of portfolio
- Identify the educational rationale for its uses
- Determine the situation where portfolio is appropriate
- Review the process of portfolio development

What is a Portfolio?

A portfolio is a repository of one's personal and professional goals, achievements, and the methods of achieving those goals. According to Hall, 'A professional portfolio is a collection of materials made by a professional that records and reflects key events, learning experiences, and processes in that professional career.' The collection not only represents the pertinent events and experiences but includes systematic and logical analysis and interpretation of those events that bring meaning to the overall process and help the individual to further his learning.

The hall-mark of portfolio as an educational process is incorporation of *goal-setting* and *self-reflection*. Goal-setting in portfolio, in contrast to other educational processes, is learner initiated and determined. Faculty often helps the learner in developing goals and may incorporate the goals and objectives of the program.

As reflection is an important concept in personal development and especially in portfolio, we expand the idea further. Reflection, in the context of educational process, is a *deliberate* and *purposeful* activity. The individual embarks on self-discovery and analysis of deciding moments in teaching and learning activities in order to learn. Thus, 'Reflection relates to a complex and deliberate process of thinking about and interpreting experience, either demanding or rewarding, in order to learn from it.' (Atkins and Murphy, 1995).

Reflection is a process that progresses through different stages. In the initial stage, the individual learner develops an awareness of uncomfortable feelings (usually due to new, unfamiliar, or negative situations). This leads to examination of components of the situation and exploration of alternative actions. Further reflective process helps the learner to develop a summary of outcomes of reflection or learning. In the final stage, the reflective thoughts result in actions (Atkins and Murphy, 1995).

The essential value of reflection as a learning tool is also highlighted and supported by Kolb's experiential learning. Although the process of reflection is mostly discussed as a process of *self-reflection*, the process can be greatly augmented by the support of faculty. Faculty can contribute to self-reflection of the learner by way of communicating the values and demonstrating the proper utilization of portfolio.

Goal-setting and reflection are two characteristics that distinguish portfolio from log-book and journal. A typical log-book contains a neatly organized collection of events and experiences. In log-books, the goals, requirements, and the process of achieving the target is mostly predetermined by the faculty and there is little opportunity for personal goal setting and reflection. Portfolio contains these events and experiences, but also includes learner-initiated goal-setting and reflection.

Similarly, journals may incorporate goals for personal and professional development in a systematic manner; but such journal entries are not corroborated by representative materials. *Reflective* journal entry, however, if it is done in the context of personal and professional development, is closer to the requirement of being a portfolio. In fact, such reflective journal entries may form one of many components of portfolio.

The Value of Portfolio

Educational values of portfolio are more obvious if we analyze it from two different perspectives: portfolio as a *process* and portfolio as a *product*. Both the process of developing a portfolio and the resultant product have significant beneficial effects on education (Winsor, 1998). These two, the process and product of portfolio, are equally important and somewhat interdependent. A good process of portfolio development ensures high quality of the final representation of the materials.

Portfolio as process

As a process, portfolio enhances the *learning* and can be used as a *self and collaborative assessment* tool. The process of portfolio development is a powerful learning process by itself—engaging the learner in the continuous process of goal setting, self-discovery and self-reflection. This is a somewhat repetitious process where the learner, with the help of faculty or teachers, identifies the priorities and decides on the goals. Over time, however, he deeply engages himself in discovery and reflection and monitors his professional and personal development.

- *Self-assessment*: Central to the development of portfolio is the ability to set individual goals and self-reflection. Portfolio encourages self-assessment by identifying what has been achieved so far, the relative efficacy and utility of various approaches to achieve the goals, and what is needed to be done in future to maximize personal and professional development.
- *Collaborative assessment*: Collaborative assessment takes place jointly by learners and teachers. Unlike other assessment methods, where teachers solely perform assessment, the portfolio provides an opportunity for joint assessment.
- *Documentation of progression of personal and professional achievements*: As the portfolio captures the key events, it helps the learner to conveniently judge the progress he has made over the course of time. Appreciation of one's own personal achievement is an effective motivational factor for continuing advancement.

In the process of portfolio development the individual does not merely collect and collate representative materials. He also determines and sets the goals of his development, documents those goals, and decides what evidence and artifacts need to be included to collaborate his progression. Moreover, he also engages in an intellectual exercise of priority setting and negotiation. Portfolio, when it is developed and maintained throughout the professional career, forms a baseline for monitoring career progression throughout the span of professional life.

The philosophy and the process of portfolio support self-directed learning, continuing and life-long learning. These are also the attributes that are most likely to succeed with adult learners.

Portfolio as product

The product of portfolio is the representative collection and documentation of the individual's attempts at self-fulfillment and development. Besides documenting what has been achieved and for what purposes, it gives an enormous sense of self-satisfaction and feeling of achievement. This also constitutes a good reference point for individual learners to communicate a chronicle of their professional development to their colleagues and mentors.

Portfolio is also used as an *assessment* instrument for students and physicians. Portfolio is designed to include artifacts such as feedback from patients, patient profile, number and nature of procedures that one performs. Such documentation, when corroborated by other performance reports, is often a requirement by the professional bodies. For example, in UK Portfolio for Pre-registration House Officers (PRHO) is promoted by General Medical Council to gather evidence of achievement of personal development plan and the Council's objectives.

As an assessment instrument, portfolio has a very significant advantage over other forms of student assessment instruments. None of the assessment instruments that we have discussed so far determine whether students or practitioners actually utilize or apply the learned knowledge in day-to-day practice. Portfolio can be designed to capture this vital piece of information. Although validity and reliability of portfolio for this specific purpose are not well established, many institutes incorporate portfolio as a student assessment instrument to collect evidence for actual transition of knowledge, attitude, and skill into practice. Similarly, professional and certifying bodies utilize portfolio as a quality assurance tool and to determine whether a certain level of competency is achieved and maintained by the practitioners.

Nature of Artifacts in Portfolio

Conceptually, the materials in portfolio belong to one of the four different types (Collins, 1991): (a) artifacts, (b) reproductions, (c) attestations, and (d) productions.

- *Artifacts:* Artifacts are materials that are produced during the course of normal work in which the learner is involved. These materials are not produced for the specific purpose of portfolio. Examples include attendance records from teaching and clinic sessions, a project or research paper that the students have written.

- *Reproductions:* Reproductions are materials, like the artifacts, that also exemplify the typical nature of work. But, unlike artifacts, these are not generally captured. Examples of reproductions include a video-recording of patient-student interactions, a video showing small group sessions that the students have conducted, or records of patients seen or procedures performed.

- *Attestations:* Attestations are, as the name implies, are materials that endorse works, efforts, and achievements. This category may include reports of students from the teachers, reports of fellow students, peer review, and letters of appreciation from patients.

- *Productions:* Productions are materials that are developed specifically for the portfolio. Examples of production include personal or professional goal statements, narratives from reflections, essays of professional and personal philosophies.

The artifacts to be included should be *representative* of the work done and do not need to be all-inclusive.

Representative Materials in Portfolio

- Goal statement
- Personal and professional philosophies
- Narratives from reflection
- Academic programs attended
- Letter of appreciation from patients
- Peer review report
- Preceptors' report
- A video recording of patient-provider interaction

Decision Making Exercise for Artifacts Inclusion

- What are the artifacts to be included?
- What are the reasons for their inclusions?
- How are they related to the decided goals?
- How much emphasis should be placed in one artifact?
- What are their comparative values?

Organization of the Portfolio

Physically, a typical portfolio is a three-ring binder that is organized into professional goals, reflection, achievements, and further goal settings. Each of these may be further compartmentalized into broad domains such as clinical experience, teaching and learning, and project and research. In the near future, personal digital assistant or similar hand-held electronic devices may replace bulky paper-based portfolio.

Organization of portfolio and materials in it closely reflects its primary purpose whether it is a learning tool or an aid to assessment. Although there is a considerable degree of latitude in deciding and choosing what to include and in what format, the decision must take into account the goal and purpose of the portfolio development. Thus, a portfolio for learning purpose should place more emphasis on the development of goal statements, reflection, self-assessment, and discovery. If portfolio is developed to aid in student assessment, more emphasis should be placed on the collection and representation of materials and records.

Organization of Professional Portfolio

- Goal statement
- Objectives
- Personal and professional philosophies
- Mentors and their role
- The process of achieving targets
- Criteria, time, frequency of assessment
- Representative artifacts: patient care, research, teaching and others
- Self-reflection and discovery
- Future plans, revised goal settings

The educational rationale of portfolio is solidly based on the philosophy of self-directed and learner-centered learning. The growing importance of the portfolio as a learning and assessment tool in medical education is the direct result of its beneficial effects on these forms of learning.

In summary, the key concepts that we have learned in the chapter are

- The portfolio is valued as a learning and assessment tool
- The critical factors of portfolio based learning are goal setting, self-reflection, and discovery
- As an educational process it supports self-directed learning, self and collaborative assessment, and progression of personal and professional achievements
- As an assessment instrument, it captures whether the learned knowledge is practiced in real life
- Content and organization of portfolio are very much dependent on the primary purpose and educational philosophies behind the development of the portfolio

References and Further Readings

1. Atkins S. and Murphy K. Reflective Practice. *Nursing Standard.* 1995. 9; 45:31–35.
2. Collins A. Portfolios for Biology Teacher Assessment. *Journal of Personnel Evaluation in Education.* 1991. 5:147–67.
3. Winsor PJT. *A Guide to the Development of Professional Portfolios in the Faculty of Education.* 1998. Faculty of Education, University of Lethbridge, Lethbridge, Alberta. Web address: http://www.edu.uleth.ca/fe/ppd/contents.html.

36 Teaching Program Evaluation

You are responsible for quality assurance in your department. Recently there has been a series of medication errors and the Head of Department requested you to design a teaching program on medication safety. The ultimate goal is to reduce the incidence of medication errors in the Department. You have conceptualized the teaching program. The curriculum consists of a combination of theories on safety, drug calculation, safe prescription techniques as well as behavioral modifications like creation of heightened awareness about safety and implementation of self-reporting of errors. You face the problem of designing a suitable evaluation tool to demonstrate the effectiveness of your effort.

Teaching program evaluation in medical education presents with a different set of challenges. The utility of such program is commonly gauged by some soft measures of outcome such as participants' general reactions about the program or the knowledge gained from it. Although these outcomes are important, we should not limit solely to these. When appropriate, we should try to judge the program's effectiveness by demonstrating that the program has resulted in real tangible benefits.

In this chapter, our tasks will be

- Discuss Kirkpatrick's program evaluation model
- Demonstrate how the model can be applied to medical education
- Cite and review examples from the model

After completing the chapter, we should develop a firm understanding of how to conduct teaching program evaluation in a structured manner.

How should we judge the effectiveness of a teaching program? What are the types of outcome parameter that we can measure? The outcome of a teaching program has several dimensions. At the simplest level, the outcome is often demonstrated by the participants' liking or disliking of the program. Other measures of success may include participants' motivation, knowledge acquisition, and transfers of knowledge into practice. In a broader sense, the ultimate outcome of a training program is something tangible and quantifiable. For example, in the above scenario the ultimate measure of success would be a reduction of department-wise medication errors or reduction in medication error related morbidity and mortality. Knowledge about all these outcomes is important for the improvement and documentation of the program's success.

Donald Kirkpatrick (1994) proposed a four-level model for training program evaluation that provides a useful and understandable structure for the educators. These levels are (a) level one: reaction, (b) level two: learning, (c) level three: transfer, and (d) level four: results. These levels are interrelated to each other and progress from a simpler level (level one: reaction) to a complex level (level four: results). Information from the prior level forms the basis of evaluation for the next level. Evaluation ideally starts at level one and, depending on available expertise and resources, advances towards higher levels. Evaluation of certain levels in isolation can be done and often practiced as well.

Level One: Reaction

Level one assesses the participants' initial reaction to a training program. The focus is on participants' immediate satisfaction and perceptions of usefulness of the program.

Advantages of level one evaluation are (a) relative ease in designing and implementing the measurement instrument, (b) ready availability of participants at the end of program, (c) utilization of the least amount of resources and money, and (d) ease in analysis. In addition, this is the only level that explicitly assesses learners' motivations and attitudes. The information from the evaluation can be utilized to improve and correct deficiencies of the program.

The major drawback is that level one only evaluates *what participants think* about the program. It is at best a measure of participants' viewpoint and may not be reflective of overall effectiveness of the program. For example, a boot camp training in the army may be perceived as too rigorous and time consuming by the trainee but its utility cannot be ignored. Despite all these drawbacks, level one is the most common assessment level that is in use in educational training. Time and resource constraints may allow only this level to be evaluated.

Both the *content* and *process* should be assessed during level one evaluation. Often times, content area receives inadequate emphasis in the evaluation instrument. Content area evaluation explores participants' reactions to materials, content coverage, and relative importance among different contents. Process area evaluation explores instructional methods such as effective use of audio-visual materials, instructional skills and enthusiasm of tutors, and facilities within the classroom. Both content and process evaluation can be used over the course of the program to determine the program's evolution and anticipated maturity.

The most common way of performing level one evaluation is to use familiar Likert's type scale where participants are asked to point out their reactions to certain statements. Level one evaluation can be done using other qualitative methods such as a focus group where the group leader elicits and probes for more specific comments about the course.

Examples of statements in Likert's scale for level one evaluation:

Process focused:

I was given sufficient information on the aims and methods of the program before my arrival.

Strongly Agree　Agree　Neutral　Disagree　Strongly Disagree

Content focused:

The materials on safe prescription habits were of good quality.

Strongly Agree　Agree　Neutral　Disagree　Strongly Disagree

Level Two: Learning

Level two assesses the amount of *information that learners have learned* from the course and thus addresses issues beyond the learners' satisfaction and attitudes. Measurement at this level is relatively more difficult and laborious. In medical education, level two evaluation assumes a significant role as knowledge acquisition is often an explicitly stated goal of a teaching program.

Although it is the cognitive (knowledge) domain that is most frequently assessed in level two evaluation, psychomotor (skill) and affective (attitude) domains can be assessed during level two evaluation as well. Assessing how well learners reconstitute and prepare appropriate medication dosages often entails significant psychomotor learning. Similarly, if the program objectives include appreciation for safe prescription writing habits then assessing how the learners' have changed their thinking would be an example of level two affective domain evaluation.

Principal pre-requisite of level two evaluation is to have a proper criterion for assessment. These are often derived from the program objectives that have been developed during the design phase of the program and constitute the benchmark against which learners are assessed.

Methods of level two assessment may include both individual and group assessment. A common example is to devise a pretest and post-test and demonstrate any change in learning before and after the program. Evaluation can be done immediately or within a short period after completion of the program.

Level Three: Transfer

Level three assesses *transfer of knowledge, skills or behavior* that has been offered in the training program to actual real life. This assessment is based on the training program objectives as well. For example, after teaching safe prescription writing, as a program evaluator, we might be interested in finding what proportion of the learners are consistently compliant with the recommendations. Thus, level three evaluation in effect assesses the strength of the program.

The tools for the assessment include observations, chart reviews (as in this example), surveys, and interviews with colleagues and fellow workers. Timing of the assessment varies but usually it is done between six weeks to six months after the end of the program. Program evaluator might also consider a follow-up evaluation to assess whether participants are still practicing those prescribed recommendations.

Level Four: Results

Level four assesses the *ultimate result of the training program.* Examples of level four evaluation include the impact of the training program in reducing cost of hospitalization for a specific condition, increasing compliance with childhood vaccination, or preventing accidental falls in a nursing home.

Level four is the most difficult level to measure. In order to be successful, it needs meticulous planning, a proper methodology of measurement, and perhaps most importantly, determination of specific objectives that the training program are expected to achieve. An explicitly stated criterion—'This program will reduce the incidence of medication errors in the department by 30% compared to baseline during the six months period following program implementation' will definitely make outcome assessment easier. Commonly used tools during level four evaluation include auditing, chart reviews, and surveys. The timing of evaluation depends on the context of training program. Despite all the difficulties and resource intensive processes, a good training program should include level four evaluation to document its real worthiness.

Table 1. Kirkpatrick's four levels of program evaluation.

Evaluation Level	What Does it Test?	Examples of Instruments
Level One: Reaction	• Participants' immediate satisfaction • Perception of usefulness • Motivation	• Likert's scale • Focus group • Structured interviews
Level Two: Learning	• Acquisition of knowledge, skills, and behavior	• Pre and post test • Standard MCQ • Essay question
Level Three: Transfer	• Transfer of knowledge, skills, and behavior into real life	• Chart-reviews • Survey • Observations
Level Four: Results	• Ultimate and intended outcome	• Chart-reviews • Survey

The correlation between all these levels may be variable. A good evaluation in level one does not necessarily translate into higher knowledge or skills acquisition in level two. Conversely, participants may evaluate a program poorly during level one but demonstrate acquisition of desired skills in level two. Nevertheless, good evaluations in level one, two, and three increase the probability of getting positive program impact during level four evaluation.

Information from program evaluation is valuable in program development and improvement. Such information also helps in program expansion, modification, and validation.

In summary, the key points that we have learned are

- Teaching program evaluation can be conveniently structured in four levels: reaction, learning, transfer, and results
- Each of these levels evaluates specific elements of the program
- An ideal program evaluation planning incorporates elements from each of these levels

References and Further Readings

1. Kirkpartick DL. *Evaluating Training Programs: The Four Level.* 1998, Second Edition. Berret Koehler Publisher.
2. Hutchinson L. Evaluating and Researching the Effectiveness of Educational Interventions. *BMJ.* 1999. 318 (5): 1267–8.
3. Wilkes M, and Bligh J. Evaluating Educational Interventions. *BMJ.* 1999. 318 (5): 1269–72.
4. Anderson SB, and Ball S. *The Profession and Practice of Program Evaluation.* 1978. Jossey-Bass. San Francisco. USA.

Section 10

Internet and Medical Education

37 Internet and Medical Education

Information technology—the internet, for example—only gives us access to information. To understand that information requires knowledge. Applying that knowledge ethically requires wisdom.

Senior Minister Lee Kuan Yew, Singapore

The wide use of the internet and e-learning has opened up remarkable opportunities for medical educators. Potential applications for e-learning in medical education can range from content development and delivery to student assessment. Increasingly, it is realized that e-learning and learner-centered and self-directed learning models can be in synergistic relationship in medical education.

In this brief chapter, our tasks are to

- Identify features of e-learning as applied to learner-centered learning model
- Determine the promises and potentials of e-learning
- Discuss basic features in designing e-learning modules

We will not deal with technical issues. After completion of this chapter, we should be able to develop a better perspective on e-learning and judiciously combine sound educational principles into e-learning to further improve learner-centered learning models.

What is E-Learning?

Electronic learning or e-learning, as it is better known, is a merger of educational process with electronic technology with the aim of bringing efficiency and effectiveness to teaching and learning.

The learning component of e-learning is usually developed from conventional teaching content with appropriate modifications to make it better suited for electronic medium. Educational concepts and principles that we have discussed in earlier chapters hold true for e-learning as well. Thus, the contents that are developed with sound educational principles in mind have a better chance of success.

The promise of the internet

- To center learning around the student instead of the classroom
- To focus on the strengths and needs of individual learners
- To make lifelong learning practical reality

The Power of the Internet for Learning; Report of the Web-Based Education Commission to the President and the Congress of the United States

---

E-learning in Learner-Centered Learning Models

As we strive towards learner-centered and self-directed learning models, several key questions naturally surface. What are the features of e-learning? What are the attributes of e-learning that make such form of learning attractive to medical educators? Can e-learning be matched harmoniously with the learner-centered learning model?

Before we answer these crucial questions we need to emphasize that e-learning, just like any educational or commercial pursuits, is prone to be influenced by many factors. Not every e-learning activity promises to be an effective one. Many e-learning ventures are mere content delivery vehicle that use electronic media for ease of delivery. Our focus here is what an *ideal* e-learning platform can provide to the learners and the promises that it holds.

As discussed in learner-centered learning model, learning is a self and collaborative activity with support and direction from the teachers and faculty. Learning is initiated and maintained by the learner, who takes up the responsibility of determining his own learning objectives, selects the learning materials and methods of learning, and takes substantial control over the monitoring of progress of learning. The learner decides what is most important for him to learn and how to carry out his own learning activities. Accordingly, a successful learner- centered learning model provides a balance between independence and support.

In most of the teacher-dominated and traditional model of learning, there is little autonomy for the learners to choose the topic of learning let alone to decide the learning objectives, methods, and materials. Teachers provide the content, usually in the form of lecture that directs to the *group* rather than individual learner with little option given to the learner. In other words, the educational activity is synchronous and insensitive to individual learner's needs and preferences [Fig. 1(a)].

E-learning model is especially attractive to medical educators as it promises to overcome the ills of teacher-dominated teaching methods by allowing learners the option of selecting learning materials in their own time and in their own preferred way. They can access the content any time and repeat the lesions as necessary from their preferred location. They can also make use of *a range of learning activities* that best suit their needs and preference. They are also able to monitor their progress and determine the success of their learning endeavors [Fig. 1(b)].

Let us critically review a model of e-learning that is based on the principles of learner-centered learning model and illustrate how the

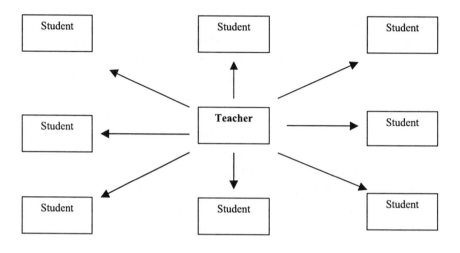

Fig. 1(a). Teacher-centered model.

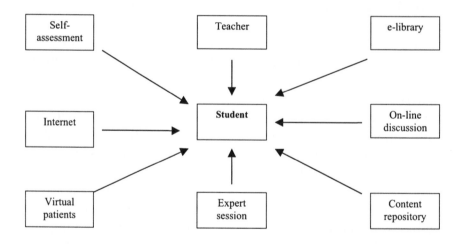

Fig. 1(b). Learner-centeredness in e-learning.

pedagogy and technology can unite in a meaningful relationship (Fig. 2). In this model, an individual learner decides to embark on a learning activity. He determines the most important priority area of his learning by taking a pre-assessment test. He gets a personalized learning plan that highlights his strengths and weaknesses in the topic and suggests several learning methods. He then engages himself in an *interactive* learning process that is *supported* by a range of learning activities and options including discussion group, e-library, expert session, practice assignment, and external link. Once he is satisfied with the learning activities he decides to test his newly acquired knowledge from online learning self-assessment. He has an option to appear for a mock test. He gets a customized achievement report with recommendations for future learning.

Several important features of this model are worth further elaboration. Firstly, the learner is able to perform a need assessment on his own to identify the priority area of study. Secondly, he is not limited to one single learning activity; rather he has the option of choosing one or several learning activities like the interactive patients, e-library, and practice assignment. Thirdly, he has the option of self-evaluating his progress and changing strategies of learning as necessary. Fourthly, the learning is supported; he is not left alone in his pursuit of learning. He has tutor and other form of support available to him. Fifthly, most of the activities can be delivered in real-time and can be accessed from many places. Finally, he has the opportunity of collaborative and social learning in the form of peer- and tutor-supported discussion with the potential of creating a virtual community of learners.

Features of e-learning in learner-centered learning

- Personalized learning plan
- Supported learning
- Promotion of collaborative and group learning
- Opportunity for self-assessment and monitoring of progress
- Variation in learning activities
- Real-time operation
- Improved access

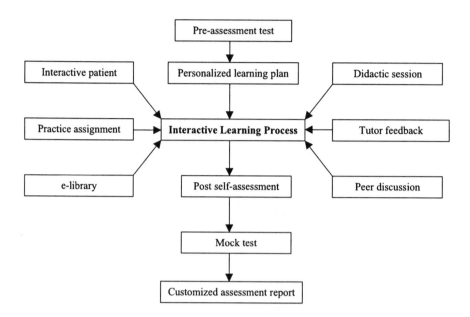

Fig. 2. Individualized learning in e-learning environment.

Design Considerations in E-Learning

The omnipresence of internet and electronic media poses many challenges and opportunities for medical educators to better design their contents and instructional methods. Technology allows interconnectivity between the content, easier access, superior and faster search ability, provision of multiple learning methods simultaneously, and support of collaborative learning. A course can be designed in such a way that the content is delivered in the form of expository text, interactive text, image-rich text, or any of these combinations.

The challenges are to convert the print and non-print content to electronic format and conversion of bulk contents, sometimes over several hundred pages, to more manageable smaller units. A lengthy learning module would be too cumbersome for the learner to browse and navigate. The developer of the course, the teacher, may also find it very difficult to update and modify the content as these involve tedious tasks of changing the entire format.

Learning Objects in E-Learning Models

To overcome the above mentioned problems and to take advantages of the best features of electronic media, the content development and delivery in e-learning are often redesigned in the form of 'learning objects'. Learning objects are 'any digital resource that can be used to support learning.' The main idea is 'to break the educational content down into small chunks that can be reused in various learning environments.' (Wiley, 2000). Learning objects, not to be confused with learning objectives, are preferred by many as a convenient and efficacious instructional strategy to develop, deliver, and manage learning in electronic media.

The elements that are incorporated in the learning objects depend on the needs and objectives of the course. It may include description of the content, learning objectives, contents, an assessment plan, and internal and external links. The learning objects also contain a structured description or meta-data that allows the content to be found easily by search.

The advantages of creating such smaller and more manageable chunks are many. By breaking down the large content into smaller components, different parts can be developed and maintained independently. Several teachers may form a group to work simultaneously and independently to develop the content. It also reduces unnecessary duplication because a well-developed learning object that is already in existence needs not be reproduced. All these factors reduce the human and financial resources for the development and maintenance of the content.

Learning objects also fit nicely into contemporary philosophy of curriculum planning that emphasizes reduction of the content load for the learners and minimization of duplication of their learning effort. For example, a learning object on diabetic medications that is used in pharmacology can be utilized during clinical years. Learning objects also bring variations in learning methods and provide learners with greater choice.

The learning object, besides being smaller in size, also needs to have several other features to make it more dynamic and educationally meaningful.

- *Self-contained*: Learning objects contain all the major components that are necessary to carry out the learning independently. Typically, such learning objects contain description of the contents, learning objectives, the actual contents, assessment plans, internal and external links.
- *Non-sequential*: The learning objects are stand-alone component that are able to meet the learning needs of the learner independently. It may not be necessary for the learner to read any other learning objects.
- *Can be aggregated*: The learning objects can be combined together into larger contents. When several of the learning objectives are grouped, they provide a comprehensive representation of the topic of interest and can be modeled into course format.
- *Reusable*: Learning objects are easily portable and can be used for multiple contents and different purposes. A learning object that is developed for a specific topic can be used in other contexts. For this characteristic, the learning objects are also known as Reusable Learning Objects (RLO).
- *Shareable:* Learning objects are also shareable between different courses, across departments, and across institutes. It is possible to create a common pool of the state-of-the-art learning objects that are shared among geographically diverse locations.

Let us consider an example to illustrate how the learning objects can be used in our context. Suppose we are given the task of creating a learning module on diabetes mellitus. This large topic can be broken down into many component parts such as physiology of glucose metabolism, disease mechanism, pharmaco-therapy, nutrition and dietary intervention, and complications. Based on this, several self-contained learning objects can be created. The content of the learning objects may incorporate lecture note, pathological slides, graphics, and clinical photographs. A learner, who is already well-familiar with physiology, may escape the learning object on physiology and move on to the ones that he needs to learn. Although each of the learning objects can stand alone, when they are combined together they would provide a broad picture of the topic. Each of the learning objects can be reused in different contexts and in different courses and thereby minimizing duplications. They can also be shared across departments and institutes.

The meteoritic rise and equally precipitous fall of e-business companies in the last decade teach us very significant lesions. The successful e-business companies are built on strong business fundamentals. They never sacrificed their business fundamentals for ease of technological wizardry. They have used technology to bolster their existing strong business foundation. Conversely, the companies that have placed technology ahead of business fundamentals perished rapidly.

If we are to extrapolate the experience of e-business, we can confidently infer that the success of the e-learning would depend upon *prudent application of technology on sound educational principles.* The factors that would determine the success of e-learning are the quality of the contents and soundness of the educational planning. The technology would make those more effective and efficient, but will not replace.

In summary, important points that we have learned are

- E-learning promises harmonious marriage with learner-centered learning models
- E-learning is supported and delivers multitudes of synchronous and asynchronous learning activities
- E-learning also encourages and promotes collaborative and group learning by creation of virtual community of learners
- Learning objects are smaller and more manageable self-contained components of a large content and one of the preferred methods of curriculum planning in e-learning
- Learning objects are reusable and shareable; they minimize duplication and redundancy in curriculum structures

References and Further Readings

1. Beck RJ. *Learning Objects*. Center for International Education. University of Milwaukee. Web address: www.uwm.edu/Dept /CIE; accessed on August 02.
2. Longmire W. *A Primer on Learning Objects*. Learning Circuits. Web address: www.learningcircuits.org; accessed on August 02.
3. *The Power of the Internet for Learning*. Report of the Web-Based Education Commission to the President and the Congress of the United States of America. December 2002. Washington DC. USA.
4. Wiley DA. Connecting Learning Objects to Instructional Design Theory: A Definition, A Metaphor, and A Taxonomy. 2000. *The Instructional Use of Learning Objects* (On-line version). Web address: http://reusability.org/read/chapters/wiley.doc; accessed August 02.

Research in Medical Education

38 Research in Medical Education

There is a widely held view among clinicians, medical researchers and medical teachers that evidence to support (or reject) educational approaches is not available. This may be true in some areas but not in others. In the area of teaching and learning communication skills in medicine, Aspergen (1999) identified 180 pertinent papers including 31 randomized studies.

R.M. Harden *et al*, 1999

It would be naïve to assume that our understanding of medical education has reached a plateau phase and we know everything that we need to know about teaching and learning in medicine. Just as medical research, medical education progresses with the generation of executable ideas, creation of working hypothesis, and testing and retesting the hypothesis to prove its worth. We are still at the formative phase of medical education research and our knowledge is evolving. As expected, the more we know about medical education, the more we will identify new issues that have not been addressed previously. The need for rigorous research is even more crucial than ever before.

In this chapter, our tasks are to

- Identify the nature of research in the context of medical education
- Propose a framework for research in medical education
- Discuss how major research initiatives have benefited medical education
- Identify selected priority areas in medical education research

Besides orienting the readers to broad and emerging fields of research in medical education, this chapter also provides insights into the similarities and differences between pure biomedical research and medical education research. We will focus more on descriptive and qualitative research for two basic reasons: (a) we are less familiar with these forms of research, and (b) they are very valuable in educational research.

Nature of Research in Medical Education

Medical education research bears many similarities with the more familiar biomedical research. The concepts and principles of research are equally applicable to medical education. Thus, the fundamental steps of hypothesis generation, random and equal allocation of subjects, reduction of variability between the groups, blinded observation, uniform outcomes measures, and sound statistical analysis are much sought after and implemented in medical educational research whenever possible.

Like biomedical research, the three broad methodological categories of medical education research are: (a) observational and descriptive, (b) co-relational, and (c) experimental. Descriptive research usually involves observation and data collection about study subjects in their natural state without any intended or unintended intervention. Co-relational research seeks to determine the relationship between outcome variables and specific groups. The intervention is unintended and allocation is non-random. Experimental research, the highest echelon of biomedical research, involves some kind of standardized intervention that is 'administered' to the group. Ideally, the allocation of study subjects to a group is random and the subject and evaluator of the results are blind.

Observational and descriptive research

An observational study often capitalizes on the examination of study subjects in their *natural* environment without any intervention and artificial restraint. The benefits of observing subjects in their natural state are well-recognized. Humans act and behave differently when they realize they are being observed. The naturalist and animal conservation scientists are acutely aware of the fact and frequently apply similar approach in observing animals in the wild. Observational study may also involve survey, interviews, audio-video recording and others.

Data from the observational study can be qualitative, quantitative or semi-quantitative. A good example of qualitative research in medical education comes from seminal research by Irby (Irby, 1994). The primary research question was to identify the components of knowledge that effective teachers in medicine need to have. The author *observed* six distinguished clinical teachers in medicine and identified six domains of knowledge essential to teaching excellence: knowledge of subject matter, knowledge of learners, knowledge of general principles of teaching and learning, and knowledge about the content specific instruction. What was impressive about the findings is the remarkable congruence among these distinguished teachers and it is reasonable to conclude that other effective clinical teachers would share the same knowledge. The findings of the research also allowed the author to propose a framework of medical teacher's knowledge.

An example of descriptive research with quantitative data comes from Amin (Amin, 2000). The author studied the recent graduates of National University of Singapore in order to identify their learning preferences. The author used Rezler's Learning Preference Inventory and determined that a very high proportion of subjects preferred concrete learning over abstract learning. There was no statistical difference between respondents' preference between teacher-centered and student-centered and between interpersonal and independent categories. The findings from the study are similar to other studies enhancing its validity.

Observational studies are valuable in exploring multiple aspects of human nature such as reaction, emotion, preferences and other forms of subjective variables. A naturalistic approach is preferred if the trait under study is susceptible to observation and other form of intrusion. In medical education, observational and descriptive research are widely practiced to explore learners' preference, characteristics of group interactions, determination of effective teaching traits, and assessing the applicability of particular learning theories.

Co-relational research

Co-relational research attempts to establish a relationship between observed outcome differences among two or more groups of study subjects. The conditions under which the two groups operate are different; but there is no proper randomization. Although the strength of evidence from co-relational research is not as robust as randomized control trials, this research does provide quality data. Frequently, the nature of the study may not allow any random allocation and blinding.

Weinholtz *et al* studied correlation between clinical teachers' behavior and learners' rating of teaching effectiveness (Weinholtz,1986). They have found that elements of teaching behavior (e.g. questioning and assessing) vary with many factors including educational level of learners, context of teaching (e.g. interview, examination, patient presentation, and discussion) and site of the teaching (bedside, hallway, and conference room). The study is important in demonstrating that learners' rating of teaching effectiveness is not unyielding and depends on many contextual variables.

Experimental research

The key component of experimental research is the deliberate administration of an intervention to the study group. In educational research such intervention commonly entails a teaching or learning program either applied to the teachers or the students. Examples of such intervention are a communication skill course to determine whether the students are better communicators after attending the course and an interactive lecture to document whether the format results in better reasoning skills among the students.

To illustrate further let us consider the following example. Jozefowicz *et al* studied the quality of in-house multiple choice questions from three US medical schools (Jozefowicz *et al*, 2002). The authors employed blind raters to assess the quality of the questions. Questions written by examiners without formal training in test writing were of poorer quality compared to questions written by examiners with formal training in test writing. The authors drew the valid conclusion that the quality of in-house examination can be significantly improved by providing question writers with formal training.

Proper randomized control trials, a form of experimental research, in medical education are comparatively fewer in number than clinical research. Nevertheless, RCT in medical education is practiced and promoted although double-blind observation is almost impossible to attain for reasons that are discussed later.

Difficulties with Interventional Research

Experimental and interventional research, although ideal, is inherently difficult to conduct in medical education. There are several practical and valid reasons for this difficulty (Norman and Schmidt, 2000; Norman, 2002). Firstly, the hard measure of evidence that we are familiar with (e.g. morbidity or mortality rate) is lacking in education. Hard measures that are available in medical education (marks in examination, pass or fail rate) are at best surrogate evidence of real outcome. Secondly, proper randomization and double blinding are challenging to practice as both the provider of the therapy (teacher) and subjects (students) are intelligent enough to recognize the intervention. Perhaps, more importantly such interventions are ethically debatable. Thirdly, it is difficult to achieve standardization in educational interventions (e.g. curricular innovations, new instructional strategy); there is no fixed dose for such interventions (Norman, 2002). Fourthly, effects of educational interventions are easy to be diluted. Students are intelligent enough to recognize the weakness of their education and resort to alternate methods to rectify the deficiencies. Also, as teaching and learning involves simultaneous practice of many varied type of activities (self-study, group discussion, tutorial), it is impossible to separate the effects of one particular educational activity from myriads of other educational activities.

Value of Qualitative Studies

One of the strategies to overcome these problems is to rely on qualitative research methodologies. Educational research literature is full of rich variety of qualitative or semi-qualitative research. Physicians, who are mostly used to quantitative studies, are generally reluctant to give credence to qualitative studies. Fortunately this is changing for the better. Detailed discussion on the properties and methodologies of qualitative research is beyond our scope. Nevertheless, there are several important considerations worth mentioning.

Qualitative research in medical education is a *valid and acceptable* way of conducting research. The data from qualitative studies often build up the conceptual framework, hypothesis generation, and solidify the theoretical underpinnings that are further studied and validated by quantitative methods. Perhaps most importantly, there are certain aspects of educational research that cannot be studied by quantitative studies. In such a situation qualitative study is not merely a valid alternative; rather it is *the methodology of choice*. For example, naturalistic observation entails observation of the subjects in their natural environment with minimum interventions. Such un-intrusive approach is invaluable in identifying learning traits and preferences and group dynamics that would not have been otherwise possible. In future, we expect to see many innovative high quality qualitative researches in medical education.

Secondary Researches in Medical Education

Apart from the primary quantitative and qualitative research, secondary research, such as systematic review and meta-analysis, has a prominent role in medical education. Systematic reviews have a special role in medical education as proper randomized control trials with single research question have not reached a critical level yet to merit a meta-analysis.

Systematic reviews are conducted in medical education to determine the current status of knowledge about a subject, consolidate findings from completed research to draw valid conclusion, develop concepts and theoretical framework, and identify the knowledge gap. Another factor that favors systematic review in medical education is that the information from qualitative studies cannot be fitted into meta-analytic model and systematic review provides a nice avenue for consolidation and inference.

The methodological principles of systematic review in medical education adhere to stringent criteria including development of valid research question, sound standard for literature search and information filtering, and valid framework for consolidation of filtered information into results. The process of systematic review can be simplified and structured. This usually begins with identifying a topic that is 'ripe' for review i.e. there is enough interest in the topic and a diverse research available in sufficient number to merit a review. Next, a thorough reading is done and expert opinions are sought to identify the key issues that would be of interest to medical educators. This leads to generation of a few, usually three to five, research questions. The next step is to read all the articles and mark the sections of the articles that are related to each of the research question. The sections are collated together under each research question to create a 'library'. The collated information is scrutinized further and eventually synthesized to create a meaningful answer for each research question (Amin *et al*, 2000; Gordon, 1993).

Amin *et al* conducted a systematic review to consolidate the research findings of three decades on 'morning report'—a form of case-based discussion of new admission cases that are practiced universally in North American residency programs. They followed the above steps and identified three key questions: (a) the purpose of morning report, (b) the teaching and learning methods during morning report, and (c) the educational benefits from such intervention. The review allowed the authors to answer the questions and provided them with substantial insights into the educational process in morning report. Equipped with these insights and after examining the examples of more promising interventions, the authors proposed a framework for morning report that would be likely to bring better educational outcomes (Amin *et al*, 2000). This example illustrates how the scope of secondary research is expanded to include practical recommendations to improve the educational process.

The utility of meta-analysis is unquestionable but the results are restrained by marked variations in almost all aspects of research including research questions, population, interventions, and outcomes. In medical education research such variability is even more striking and as expected, there are very few meta-analyses.

Framework for Research

How do we establish a relationship between qualitative, interventional, randomized control, and secondary researches? How does the research progress in medical education? Let us consider a hypothetical situation; we are to embark on a research to determine whether training the teachers on bedside teaching results in better educational outcomes in the students. We face an immediate problem of determining the nature of clinical teaching. Is it a homogenous entity with every teacher following the same teaching method? Or, is it a combination of wide ranging teaching activity? Answers to these questions most likely would come from some form of observational studies; perhaps clandestine and unobtrusive video recordings of clinical teaching. Unless we know about these preliminaries, it would be impossible to agree upon a particular type of educational intervention that we may want our teachers to be trained on. The qualitative study would be likely to determine varied teaching activities (e.g. directive, question and answer format, practical hands on demonstration) that are employed by the teachers.

The next stage would involve identifying the teaching activity, either in isolation or in combination, which holds the promise to be successful. Evidence for this would come from comparisons of relative effectiveness between teachers who consistently practice one modality of teaching. For example, teacher A consistently practices the didactic method while teacher B consistently practices question and answer format during clinical teaching. A co-relational study to document the educational outcomes between the students of teacher A and teacher B would help us to identify which of the educational activities, didactic or question and answer format, is more successful. Suppose, we find that question and answer format results in superior outcome. The final evidence would come from a randomized trial with an intervention in the form of training the teachers on proper question and answering technique.

This simplified model illustrates how the educational research may progress. Qualitative studies are imperative in new situations to understand educational processes and to generate credible hypotheses. A co-relational study provides support in favor of one intervention over the others and is helpful in situations where a randomized trial is still premature or not pragmatic. The final evidence comes from randomized control and other forms of interventional trial. A systematic review consolidates the existing findings, proposes new concepts and theories, and identifies new research questions based on existing literature.

Priority Research Areas in Medical Education

Priority research areas in medical education are many and depend on the needs and the mission of individual institutes. Need-based research is a pragmatic approach for a budding medical education researcher or for a newly established medical education unit. Whereas hypothetical or theory-based research is more appropriate for mature researcher and established medical education units.

Need-based research directly answers the questions related to individual or institutional needs and is of immediate interest to the faculty and the administrators. Funding and other administrative support for such research is easier to secure as the research directly contributes to institutional development.

The foundation and theoretical modeling of such research is already in existence in the literature. A new researcher may not need to invest valuable resources and time to develop an entirely new theoretical framework. Similarly, if the research demands comparison with other educational models, it is likely that such models are already in existence. Examples of need-based research include creation of learning profiles of the students, establishing the relationship between students' admission scores and the final outcome, demonstrating the effectiveness of a new teaching module, and comparisons of students in two different curricular models.

Collaboration in Medical Education Research

The prolific and ever expanding nature of medical education research speaks for the creation of a common repository of research literature for ease of access and dissemination. Best Evidence Medical Education (http://www.bemecollaboration.org/) is an initiative that has been undertaken to collect and review best evidences and research findings in medical education. The proposed Medical Education Outcome Commission envisions creation of a repository for measures and instruments that would also provide uniform recommendations to conduct quality studies with measurement instruments (Bordage *et al*, 1998).

The research in medical education has contributed significantly in our understandings of teaching and learning in medicine. Medical education research is not merely academic and esoteric in nature. On the contrary, the vast majority of the studies and publications address issues that are practical and of immediate interest to medical teachers.

In summary, important points that we have learned are

- Research in medical education is generally similar to biomedical research with few notable differences
- Qualitative research is valid and useful in examining new issues, generating range of hypotheses, and proposing newer concepts and premises
- Interventional study with randomization and double-blinding is difficult to achieve in educational research
- Systematic reviews consolidate qualitative or semi-quantitative data and effective in dealing with heterogeneous researches
- Need-based research is more feasible and fitting for budding individuals and medical education units

References and Further Readings

1. Amin Z. How Do Our New Graduates Prefer to Learn. *Singapore Medical Journal*. 2000. 41(7): 317–23.
2. Amin Z, Guajardo J, Wisniewski M, Bordage G, Tekian A, and Niederman LG. Morning Report: Focus and Methods Over the Past Three Decades. *Academic Medicine*. 2000. 75 (10 supplement): S1–5.
3. Bordage G, Burack JH, Irby DM, and Stritter FT. Education in Ambulatory Settings: Developing Valid Measures of Educational Outcomes, and Other Research Priorities. *Academic Medicine*. 1998. 73(7): 743–50.
4. Gordon MJ. Organizing and Managing an Interactive Review of Literature. Seattle, WA: Department of Family Medicine. School of Medicine. University of Washington. 1993.
5. Harden RM, Grant J, Buckley G, and Hart IR. BEME Guide No. 1: Best Evidence Medical Education. *Medical Teacher*. 1999. 21 (6): 553–62.

6. Irby DM. What Clinical Teachers in Medicine Need to Know? *Academic Medicine*. 1994. 69(5): 333–42.
7. Jozefowicz RF *et al.* The Quality of In-house Examinations. *Academic Medicine*. 2002. 77(2): 156–61.
8. Norman G, and Schmidt HG. Effectiveness of Problem-Based Learning Curricula: Theory, Practice and Paper Darts. *Medical Education*. 2000. 34: 721–8.
9. Norman G. Research in Medical Education: Three Decades of Progress. *British Medical Journal*. 2002. 324: 1560–2.
10. Weinholtz D, Albanese M, Zeitler R, Everett G, and Shymansky J. Effective Attending Physician Teaching: The Correlation of Observed Instructional Activities and Learner Rating of Teaching Effectiveness. *Proc Annu Conf Res Med Educ*. 1986. 25: 273–8.

Appendix A

Calgary-Cambridge Observation Guide

Calgary-Cambridge Observation Guide is an actual example of communication skill training session that has been well-validated and widely used. Calgary-Cambridge Observation Guide divides communication in medical settings into two broad categories: (a) interviewing the patient and (b) explanation and planning. Each of the categories has several components. For example, interviewing the patient is further divided into (a) initiating the session, (b) gathering information, (c) building relationship, and (d) explaining and planning.

Several features of the observation guides are noteworthy. First, the guide is need-based; the sessions are structured according to need of the moments. Therefore there are separate guide for 'Interview' and 'Explanation and Planning'. Second, the sessions progress sequentially from one part to another. Finally, these guides can be used as checklists for assessment and to provide feedback to the learners.

Calgary-Cambridge Observation Guide One
Interviewing the Patients

Initiating the session

1. Greets patient and obtains patient's name
2. Introduces self and clarifies role
3. Demonstrates interest and respect, attends to physical comfort
4. Identifies and confirms patient's problem list or issues
5. Negotiates agenda: taking both patient's and doctor's perspective into account

Gathering information

Exploration of problems

6. Encourages patient to tell story
7. Appropriately moves from open to closed questions
8. Listens attentively
9. Facilitates patient's responses verbally and non-verbally
10. Uses concise, easily understood questions and comments
11. Clarifies patient's statements
12. Establishes dates

Understanding the patient agenda

13. Determines and acknowledges patient's ideas
14. Explores concern
15. Determines patient's expectations for each problem
16. Encourages expression of feeling and thought
17. Picks up verbal and non-verbal clue

Structuring the consultation

18. Summarizes at end of specific line of inquiry
19. Progresses from one section to another using transitional statements
20. Structures interview in logical sequences
21. Attends to timing and keeping interview on task

Building relationship

22. Demonstrates appropriate non-verbal behavior
23. If reads, writes notes or uses computer does in a manner that does not interfere with dialogue or rapport
24. Accepts legitimacy of patient's view and non-judgmental
25. Empathizes with and supports patient
26. Deals sensitively with embarrassing and disturbing topics and physical pain
27. Appears confident and reasonably relaxed
28. Shares thinking with patient when appropriate to encourage patient's involvement

Explaining and planning: closing the session

29. Gives explanations at appropriate time
30. Gives information in clear, well-organized, complete fashion without overloading patient
31. Checks patient's understanding and acceptance of explanation and plans
32. Encourages patient to discuss any additional points and provides him/her opportunity to do so
33. Closes interview by summarizing briefly, contracting with patient regarding next step for patient and physician

Calgary-Cambridge Observation Guide One
Explanation and Planning

Explanation and planning

Providing the correct amount and type of information

1. Initiates: Summarizes to date, determines expectations, and sets agenda
2. Assesses patient's starting point: asks for patient's prior knowledge early, discovers extent of patient's wish for information

3. Gives information in assimilable chunks and checks for understanding
4. Asks patient what other information would be useful
5. Gives explanation at appropriate times: avoids giving advice, information or reassurance prematurely

Aiding accurate recall and understanding

6. Organizes explanation: divides into discrete sections and develops a logical sequence
7. Uses explicit categorization and sign-posting
8. Uses repetition and summarization
9. Uses concise and easily understood statements, and avoids or explains jargon
10. Uses visual methods of conveying information: diagrams, models, written information and instructions
11. Checks patient's understanding of information given: asks patient to restate in own words; clarifies as necessary

Incorporating the patient's perspective—achieving shared understanding

12. Relates explanation to patient's illness framework
13. Provides opportunities and encourages patient to contribute
14. Picks up verbal and non-verbal clues
15. Elicits patient's beliefs, reactions and feeling

Planning shared decision making

16. Shares own thought: ideas, thought processes and dilemma
17. Involves patient by making suggestions rather than directive
18. Encourages patients to contribute their ideas, suggestions, preference, belief
19. Negotiates a mutually acceptable plan
20. Offers choices: encourages patient to make choices and decisions to level they wish

21. Checks with patient: acceptance of plan and address of concern

Options in explanation and planning

If discussing opinion and significance of problem

22. Offers opinions of what is going on
23. Reveals rationale for opinion
24. Explains causation, seriousness, expected outcome, short and long-term consequences
25. Checks patient's understandings of what has been said
26. Elicits patient's beliefs, reactions, and concerns

If negotiating mutual plan of actions

27. Discusses various options
28. Provides information on action and treatment offered: (a) name (b) steps involved and how it works, (c) benefits and disadvantages, and (d) possible side-effects
29. Elicits patient's understandings, reactions, and concerns about plans and treatment including acceptability
30. Obtains patient's view of need for actions, perceived benefits, barriers, motivation
31. Takes patient's lifestyle, belief, cultural background and abilities into consideration
32. Encourages patient to be involved in implementing plans, to take responsibilities, and be self reliant
33. Asks about patient's support systems, discusses other support available

If discussing investigation and procedures

34. Provides clear information on procedures
35. Relates procedures with treatment plan
36. Encourages questions and expression of thoughts regarding potential anxieties and negative outcome

Closing the session

37. Summarizes session briefly
38. Contracts with patient regarding next steps for patient and physicians
39. Discusses safety nets appropriately and explains possible unexpected outcome
40. Checks that patient agrees and is comfortable with plan and asks if any correction, questions or other items to discuss

(Published with permission: Kurtz S, Silverman J, and Draper J. *Teaching and Learning Communication Skills in Medicine.* *Calgary-Cambridge Observation Guide.* Appendix 2. Page 226–31. Published by Radcliffe Medical Publishers. Oxon. UK. Professor Kurtz has also given kind permission.)

Appendix B

Example of Standardized Patient Case Script

Basic Particulars

Case write-up team: John Doe MD (Clinician)
                              Mary Goh (SP Trainer)
                              Zubair Amin MD MHPE (Medical Educator)

Date: 30th September, 2002

Objectives: Approach to a patient with hypertension and cerebro-vascular accident. The students should be able to

a) Generate differential diagnosis of patient's condition by appropriate history and physical examination
b) Propose a plan of investigations
c) Suggest a plan of management appropriate for the patient
d) Demonstrate appropriate interview and counseling techniques

General instructions to the standardized patient

- Strictly adhere to the facts
- The historical or physical examination findings that are not present in the script should be taken as negative
- Do not over-dramatize
- Stay in the role from beginning to the end
- Limit to presenting complaints
- Patient should ask questions about illness, management plan, medication, and prognosis

Standardized Patient's Particulars

- Name: Adrian Tan
- Age: 45 years
- Race: Chinese
- Gender: Male
- Smoking: Occasional, half-a-pack a day
- Drinking: Social drinking only
- Medication: None on regular basis, occasionally taken blood pressure pill
- Allergy: None
- Education: Graduate
- Activity: Sedentary life style. Participate in community activities on regular basis
- Diet: Average
- Dress: In hospital gown with under-garments
- Position: Lying on the bed
- Built: Average
- Language efficiency: English and Chinese
- Other special attribute: None
- Marital status: Married with two children
- Occupation: Administrative officer
- Economic status: Middle class
- Prior medical history: Told to have high blood pressure during a health fair. Did not pursue further.

- Support system: Lives with wife; owns a HDB three bed-room apartment
- Family history: Father had a history of hypertension and died of stroke at age 66. Mother is well.

Presenting Scenario

- Settings: Accident and Emergency Room
- Chief complaint: "I don't know what happened to me. I was in my office. I had a long meeting and after that I tried to take some rest in the couch. When I tried to get-up I found I couldn't do it. After several minutes my colleagues noticed that I was not able to move my right side."

Presenting History

Onset: The onset of this episode was sudden. Patient was in the office in his couch taking some rest after a long day of work. When he wanted to get-up, he realized he could not do so. His friends helped him to get out of the couch and brought him to the A&E. His friends also noticed that he was not moving his right side. Initially Mr. Tan did not realize his weakness, although he had some funny feelings in his affected side.

Location and nature of motor impairment

Limbs:

- The right side of the body
- Both the upper and lower extremities are affected
- Weakness involves both proximal and distal muscles groups (arm, forearm, and hand)
- Unable to shrug the shoulder on the right side

Face:

- Right side of the face is weak
- When he tries to talk, the face deviates to the *left*
- When ask to protrude the tongue, it deviates to the right

The weakness is generally limited to the right side of the body and ends in the midline.

The motor strength is 2/5 on the right side both in upper and lower extremities. Patient is unable to initiate a hand-shake and when offered he lifts up the right hand with the left. He is unable to make a strong grip with right hand. The motor strength on the left side is unaffected. Facial expression suggests obvious embarrassment.

Deep tendon reflexes are diminished in the right side of the body; biceps, triceps, brachio-radialis, patellar and ankle all show diminished reflexes. The deep tendon reflexes are preserved in left-side.

Babinski's sign is positive in the right side and negative in the left side.

Eye-movement is not affected in either side

Shoulder shrug is weak on right-side

Cerebellar functions are intact on left side and unable to demonstrate on right side

Other characteristics

The impairment is unremitting in nature with no progression or improvement since the onset. There is no identifiable precipitating factor. There is no alleviating or aggravating factor. There is no radiation to other parts of the body. There is no pain. This is the first episode.

Location and nature of sensory impairment

Diminished pinprick and crude touch on right side of the body especially on right upper extremity and right trunk up to the midline. In the right lower extremity the sensation is diminished but less so than the upper extremity.

Vibration and awareness of joint movement and position are diminished on right upper extremity but preserved on the right lower extremity. Left side is unaffected.

There is diminished sensation on the right side of the face; sensation is relatively preserved on the forehead. Left side of the face is unaffected.

Body language, posture, and emotional state

- Appears sad and confused
- Sits with right shoulder lagging
- Co-operative with physicians
- Needs help in standing and ambulation
- Unable to lie-down from sitting position and sit-up from lying position without help
- Bowel and bladder function is continent but the patient is very worried about this

Memory and cognition

- Both short and long-term memory are intact
- Able to remember events in the past

Speech and language

- Lacks fluency
- Speech appears slurred
- Content of the speech is appropriate

Mental status examination

- Normal and appropriate for the situation

Other physical examinations and vitas signs (to be provided to the students)

- Heart rate: 82 beats/minute
- Respiratory rate: 16 breaths/minute
- Oxygen saturation: 98% on room air

- Blood pressure: 142/96 mm of Hg (students perform on their own.   Blood pressure reading can be manipulated by re-calibrating the machine.)
- SP will have normal respiratory, cardiac, abdomen, musculo-skeletal, and skin examination.

Appendix C

Further Resources

For the interested readers, we have compiled a list of internet resources on medical education. Access to these representative sites further directs to many other web addresses.

Professional Medical Education Organization

1. Association of American Medical Colleges;
   www.aamc.org
2. The American Board of Internal Medicine;
   www.abim.org
3. Ambulatory Pediatric Association;
   www.ambpeds.org
4. Best Evidence Medical Education;
   www.bemecolloboration.org
5. World Federation for Medical Education;
   www.sund.ku.dk/wfme
6. The Network: Towards Unity for Health;
   www.the-networktufh.org

7. The Association of Program Director in Internal Medicine; http://apdim.med.edu/
8. Royal Society for Physician and Surgeon of Canada; www.rcpsc.edu

Educational Data Bases

1. Educational Resources Information Center (ERIC); www.eric.ed.gov
2. PsycINFO; http://www.apa.org/psycinfo

Medical Education Discussion Group

1. MED-ED: List-serv system with primary interest in application of electronics in medical education. The site is maintained by AAMC.
   http://www.aamc.org/meded/software/start.htm
2. DR-ED: Listserv system maintained by OMERAD (Office of Medical Education Research and Development at Michigan State University, College of Human Medicine) as a mean of information and resource sharing for medical education. DR-ED is open to anyone involved in medical education. Messages posted to DR-ED should be limited to discussions and information related to medical education.
   Send an e-mail message to Listserv@list.msu.edu. Leave the subject line blank, and in the body of the message type: SUBSCRIBE DR-ED firstname lastname. Replace firstname lastname with your own first and last names.
   Web address: http://www.msu.edu/unit/omerad/DR-ED/
3. Problem-Based Learning:
   Send an email to listproc@sparky.uthscsa.edu with the following message 'subscribe pblist' followed by 'first name last name'

Medical Education Journals

1. Teaching and Learning in Medicine;
   http://edaff.siumed.edu/tlm/
2. Academic Medicine;
   www.academicmedicine.org
3. Medical Education;
   www.mededuc.com
4. Medical Education Online;
   www.med-ed-online.org

Faculty Development Resources

1. Center for Instructional Support;
   http://www.uchsc.edu/CIS/
2. Residents' Teaching Skill Web Site;
   http://www.ucimc.netouch.com/
3. The American College of Physician;
   http://www.acponline.org
4. University of California, Department of Education;
   http://www.gse.uci.edu/
5. University of Hawaii, Faculty Development Program;
   http://www.hawaii.edu/icmsig/learn.html#FacDev
6. IMSA Center for Learning and Instruction;
   http://www.imsa.edu/team/cpbl.htm
7. University of Delaware Problem-Based Learning;
   http://www.udel.edu/pbl/
8. Maricopa Center for Learning and Instruction;
   http://www.mcli.dist.maricopa.edu/pbl

Appendix D

Glossary of Terms

There are number of terms that are commonly used in medical education. General readers in medical education quite often find the terms difficult to understand. In this chapter we introduce selected medical education terms. The terms are selected based on their relevance and importance. Some of the terms discussed in this chapter are covered in detail in the book, while several other terms are not discussed or discussed briefly. The terms are discussed in relation to the concepts of medical education and in line with the spirit and philosophy of the book. The general educational terms are modified and concepts are simplified. When there are several definitions of the same term we have chosen the one that closely resembles the purpose of the book.

Accreditation

Accreditation is a regulatory process whereby a professional and/or governmental body assesses a particular educational institute or program to ascertain whether it has met the accepted level of standard.

Affective domain

This concerns attitude, belief, or value of a person. It is the combination of action and inclination that express our feelings towards the others. Example: attitudes towards terminally ill patients.

Aim

Aim is the final outcome that a teaching or educational program is expected to achieve.

Answer

Answer is defined as 'any response that fulfills the expectation of the question.'

Assessment

Assessment is the systematic process of making inference about the learning and development of the students. It includes ongoing or formative assessment as well as end of rotation summative assessment. Assessment is linked with learning objectives.

Basic Science Years

It is the preliminary one to two years in medical schools when basic sciences such as anatomy, physiology, and biochemistry are introduced on the assumption that they form the foundation for the future clinical years. Basic science years are also known as preclinical years. The demarcation between basic science and clinical years is criticized as being artificial and there is a greater call for integration.

Bedside Teaching

Bedside teaching refers to history taking, physical examination, and clinical reasoning exercise that are carried out with real patients. Typically the teaching takes place in the inpatient or in the ambulatory clinic beside patient's bed and under direct observation and supervision of the preceptor.

Bedside Manner

This refers to the expected professional behavior and attitude of the physician in dealing with the patient. It includes such attributes as cultural and social sensitivity, politeness, and confidentiality in dealing with patient problem.

Brainstorming

Brainstorming is an active learning strategy that capitalizes individual learner's ability to generate a range of ideas and thoughts. The brainstorming session is carried out in a group situation where the learners activate prior knowledge and work on solving a specific task or problem.

Clinical Competence

Clinical competency is a holistic and comprehensive concept that dictates the level of mastery that a medical student or a physician is required to attain to deal with clinical problems effectively. The concept encompasses various traits including knowledge, physical examination skill, data gathering, interpretation, decision-making ability, and interpersonal communications.

Cognitive Domain

This refers to 'cognition' or mental process and encompasses many traits such as knowledge acquisition, conceptualization, information processing, data analysis, and problem solving.

Competence

Competence is the *actual* attainment of requisite knowledge, attitude and behavior, and skills.

Continuing Medical/Professional Education

Continuing Medical Education or CME is a continuous process of learning and mastering new knowledge and skill throughout the entire professional career. The need for CME arises with the changing and ever expanding nature of medical knowledge and own professional demand.

Curriculum

Curriculum is the total blue-print, a comprehensive academic plan, which outlines the overall process of educational program.

The curriculum contains description of learning objectives and learning strategies to achieve those objectives, and a detailed assessment plan.

Domain

A domain of learning is the grouping of educational objectives into a distinctly limited area of knowledge (Rubenstein and Talbot, 1992). By listing the objectives into similar category, it is possible to simplify the learning tasks. For example, for a complex task such as airway intubation, all knowledge related objectives can be grouped together for ease of learning.

Educational Objectives

Educational objectives are brief description of what the learners are expected to achieve after attending an educational program. Educational objectives are also described as *learning* objectives, as opposed to teaching objectives, to emphasize that these objectives essentially describe what the learner should be able to do after the educational program.

Educational Needs

Educational needs describe the current status of the learner and represent the gap between the present knowledge and skills of the learners and where they should be at the end of the planned educational activities.

Evaluation

It is the systematic process of data collection about the educational program or activity with the aim of making better decisions. Evaluation processes include a measurement component and a judgment or decision component (Guilbert, 1981).

Facilitator

Facilitator is the preferred term to describe the 'teacher' in learner-centered learning model. The role of facilitator is to 'facilitate learning'—encourage and assist the learner to achieve the learning objectives. This is a major advancement from the traditional role of the teacher where the teacher assumes a dominant role in the education.

Faculty Development

Faculty development is a systematic process of educating teachers about the science of medical education in order to improve their teaching. As medical teachers are content expert without much knowledge about educational processes, faculty development is essential before delegating the duty of teaching to them.

Feedback

Feedback is a communication technique in which teacher provides information to students about their progress in mastering certain skills or achieving learning objectives of the course. Feedback is often viewed as a part of formative assessment process.

Flexner Report

It is one of the most significant reports on medical education that changed the landscape of medical education. In 1910, Abraham Flexner published the report 'Medical Education in the United States and the Canada'. The report, among other recommendations, suggested incorporation of biomedical science with hands-on clinical training. It also emphasized greater accountability and need for standards in medical schools.

Hybrid Curriculum

This refers to a compromised model of curriculum where PBL is practiced alongside with more traditional instructional methods.

Learning

This is a process resulting in some modifications, relatively permanent, of the way of thinking, feeling, and doing of the learner.
Characteristics of learning include

- Results in behavior change in the learner
- Leads to relatively permanent change
- Results from practice, repetitions, and experience

Learning is *not* the result of natural maturation process (Guilbert, 1981).

Learning Contract

Learning contract is a structured learning plan where the learners determine their own learning objectives, learning strategies, and assessment methods based on their own needs and experience. This is generally negotiated with and agreed upon by the faculty.

Learning Experience

Learning experience is the combination of many interconnected activities that help the learner progress towards achieving specific learning objectives. Learning experience can be varied and includes formal activities such as lecture or other informal or semi-formal activities such as self-reading, group discussion, brainstorming etc.

Learning Issues

In the context of PBL, learning issues are the most important and relevant topics that deserve further learning by the learners.

Life-Long Learning

The concept emphasizes that the training of physician only begins at medical school and continues throughout the professional career. It is the professional and moral responsibility of physician to prepare for and carrying out learning effectively beyond the medical school.

Medical Educator

Medical educators are persons with special interest and expertise in medical education. They may be physician by training or professional from other disciplines such as education, psychology, and allied health sciences.

Metacognition

Meatcognition is the *skill of learning*. It refers to a learner's awareness of objectives, ability to plan and evaluate learning strategies, and ability to monitor progress and adjust learning behavior to accommodate needs (Flavel, 1979).

Needs Assessment

Needs assessment is the systematic process of collecting data in order to define the educational needs. Needs assessment is usually carried out at the planning stage of educational activities and identifies the current status. Needs assessment may target individual learners or a program.

Organ-Based Curriculum

It is a model of curriculum that attempts to bring integration within the organ system by combining both pre-clinical and clinical disciplines. Although, the approach is deemed to be superior to fragmented curriculum, it still fails to satisfy more through integration that is favored by contemporary medical education.

Portfolio

Portfolio as a learning process is one of learning strategies of learner-centered learning. The learner is required to set own learning objectives, decides on the method to achieve the objectives, and engage in several varied learning experiences. The process emphasizes systematic collection of artifacts and objects over the period of learning to provide evidence of the learning progression. Portfolio is also used as an assessment tool with the idea of capturing what a student or practitioner actually *does* in real situation.

Problem-Based Learning

Problem based learning (PBL) is used to denote both curricular innovation as well as description of instructional model. PBL is supported by small group activity. In PBL problem is presented first, the group discusses the problem and, with the help of facilitator, identifies the learning issues. In next stage, the group reads about the learning issues and presents those to the rest. There are innumerable variations, adaptations, and innovations within the basic framework.

Professionalism

A set of core values or standards that every physician is expected to have. The values reflect the expectations of the society, professional bodies, patients, and peers. It emphasizes that the quality of a physician is not limited to knowledge but includes other humanistic qualities such as empathy, respect, humanity, and sensitivity to patients' belief system.

The components of professionalism include altruism, accountability, duty, excellence, honor and integrity, and respect for others (ABIM, Project Professionalism).

Psychomotor Domain

This is the area of learning that often involves performing certain skills that require manipulation of instruments and equipment. Examples: physical examination skills, insertion of IV canula.

Question

Question refers to anything that intends to elicit of an answer regardless of grammatical form.

Closed-ended questions require selection of limited range of choices. Open-ended questions allow much wider range of choices to select from.

Reflection

Reflection is a deliberate and purposeful process when the learner embarks on self-discovery and analysis of deciding moments in life in order to learn. Reflection is an important component in Kolb's experiential learning model.

Self-Assessment

This is the process of assessing own learning including the assessment of the effectiveness of learning strategies, outcomes, and identifying the better strategies for future usage. As an educational process, self-assessment is highly valued as this allows learners to take control of their own learning. It is an important component of self-directed learning.

Self-Directed Learning

Self-directed learning delegates the responsibility of learning to the learner. Learners identify the needs for the learning, initiate the learning process, decide on the learning objectives, determine the learning strategies to achieve the objectives, and finally plan for the assessment.

Skill

It is the ability to perform an educational task with an accepted level of standard. Although, commonly understood as motor skill, the term is used to describe psychological task (e.g. counseling skill) as well.

Small Group

Small group is formed when few (usually 5–10 learners) work together with the task of attaining common educational objectives. The learning in small group is bolstered by group interaction.

Subject-Based Curriculum

This is an antiquated curricular model where the subject is taught separately and in isolation. This model is superceded by more integrated curricular models.

Sub-Skills

This refers to the individual component of skills within a complex skill. Sub-skills are utilized to teach complex task that may be difficult for the learner to assimilate in whole. The method is used commonly for teaching counseling and complex motor task.

Teacher-Centered Education

This is a teaching philosophy where the teacher is a dominant partner in education with the role of providing instruction to the students. The learning is learner-passive and insensitive to learners' needs and preference.

Teaching

Teaching is the interaction between teacher and student under the teacher's responsibility in order to bring about expected changes in student's behavior. The purpose of teaching is to facilitate learning.

Teaching helps students
- Acquire, retain, and be able to use knowledge
- Understand, analyze, and synthesize knowledge
- Achieve skills
- Build attitudes (Guilbert, 1981)

Teaching Scripts

Teaching scripts are short clinical vignette that are highly organized and stimulus driven and contain anticipated internalized information about the learners, the goal of the session, specific teaching points for the given topics, and possible learning strategies. These teaching scripts help teachers anticipate learners' actions in advance and enable them to respond quickly during an instructional episode (Irby, 1992).

Tips on Using Technical Terms

If you intend to use these technical terms with others or during educational workshop, we suggest following tips to convey easily the underlying meaning.

- Explain that the terms are adapted to fit medical education and may not be generalized to other disciplines
- Explain the concept *first* and then use technical terms. That way, learners will be able to connect the concept with the term and less likely to be alarmed at the beginning
- Allow sufficient time for the learner to assimilate the ideas especially when using the terms for the first time
- Use simple *analogy* that the learners can easily relate to
- Encourage the learner to create a list of terms that they have encountered and set aside separate time to discuss those
- Explore the learner's understanding of the terms to get an insight about their thinking process

References and Further Readings

1. Ambulatory Pediatric Association. Web address: www.ambpeds.org; accessed June 2002.
2. Flavel JH. Metacognition and Cognitive Monitoring: A New Area of Psychological Inquiry. *American Psychologist.* 1979 (34): 906–11.
3. Guilbert J-J. *Educational Handbook for Health Personnel.* Revised Edition. 1981. World Health Organization. Geneva, Switzerland.
4. Irby D. How Attending Physicians Make Instructional Decisions When Conducting Teaching Rounds. *Academic Medicine.* 1992. (67): 630–8.
5. Rubenstein W and Talbot Y. *Medical Teaching in Ambulatory Care: A Practical Guide.* Springer Series on Medical Education. 1992. Springer. NY. USA.
6. The American Board of Internal Medicine. *Project Professionalism.* Web address: http://www.abim.org/pubs/profess.pdf. Accessed June 02.
7. Wojtczak A. Glossary of Medical Education Terms. Institute of International Medical Education. New York. USA. Web address: www.iime.org; accessed June 2002.

Index

Academic Medicine, 3, 293, 298
adult learner, 5, 41–46, 328
adult learning, 5, 35, 41–45, 50, 116
affective domain, 82, 83, 85, 86, 338, 386
analysis, 33, 78, 80, 85, 106, 107, 116, 123, 283, 284, 288–290, 314, 326, 337, 358
answer, 17, 20, 51, 70, 83, 100, 108–112, 117, 127, 129, 285, 286, 288–291, 294–296, 298, 301–306, 313, 314, 347, 363–366, 386
application of the knowledge, 78
articulation, 82
artifacts, 328–332
Asian medical schools, 15
assessment, x, xi, xiii–xv, 4, 7–10, 16, 20–22, 28, 31, 32, 34, 37, 43, 45, 46, 60–62, 64, 69–71, 76, 77, 85, 86, 90–93, 95, 119, 121, 283–285, 287, 293, 294, 298–303, 306, 309–314, 317–323, 325, 327–329, 331, 332, 337–340, 345, 348, 349, 351, 352, 386
Association of American Medical Colleges, 204
attitudes, 8, 18, 60, 61, 76, 77, 82, 86, 91, 131, 133, 296, 337, 338

audience, 256

Bangladesh, vii, 15
Barrows, Howard, 317
basic science, xii, 5, 15, 17–23, 127, 292, 293, 386
Best Evidence Medical Education, 366
Bloom's taxonomy, 75, 78
British system, 15

Calgary-Cambridge Observation Guide, 206, 369–374
case, iv, 9, 30, 38, 61, 63, 100, 101, 116, 123–130, 136, 137, 291, 293, 294, 304, 306, 312, 320–323, 364
case writing, 225
case-based teaching, 32, 103, 123–126, 129, 130
casual reasoning, 176, 177
change, v, vi, xiii, 6, 9, 13, 16, 17, 19–21, 27, 28, 37, 52, 61–66, 83, 91, 100, 106, 133, 285, 338, 339, 349
China, 15, 23
clinical competence, 310, 314, 319, 323, 387
clinical reasoning, 7, 9, 103, 310

clinical teacher, 320, 321, 359, 360
clinical teaching, xi, xiii, xiv
close-ended questions, 143
co-relational research, 358, 360
cognition, 39, 77, 81, 108, 118, 296, 387
communication skills, 18, 60, 103, 131,
    139, 311, 320, 357, 361
competency, 3, 4, 6–9, 61, 294, 311, 312,
    329
comprehension, 37, 78, 79, 85, 287, 288
Confucius, 99
conservatism, 273, 274
constructivist theory, 30, 116
criticism, 5, 17, 18, 23, 147, 154, 158,
    185
curriculum, 21, 57, 58, 62, 335, 351,
    353, 387
curriculum
    design, 5, 57, 58
    implementation, 9, 57–60, 62–66,
        243, 246

deep learning, 4, 27, 32–34, 38
deterministic reasoning, 177
difficulty index, 295
distracter, 126, 286, 287
domain, 4, 61, 75–78, 80–82, 85, 86, 94,
    102, 284, 287, 293, 310, 313, 323, 331,
    338, 359, 388
DR-ED listserv, 3, 382

e-learning, 345–351, 353
educational concepts, 27, 346
ERIC, 39, 46, 53, 112, 122, 139, 382
essay question, 299, 301–304, 306, 340
evaluation, 5, 19, 20, 22, 41, 43, 51–53,
    58, 62, 63, 69, 76–78, 80, 81, 85, 90,
    95, 284, 290, 291, 295, 296, 302, 306,
    311, 335–341
experiential learning, 4, 27, 33–38, 326
extended matching item, 285, 293

facilitator, 30, 31, 42, 388
faculty development, 21–23, 389
feedback, 30, 58, 62, 69, 101, 103, 134,
    139, 310, 311, 319, 321, 329, 389

Flexner, Abraham, 14–16, 22, 186, 389
formative assessment, 183, 252, 257,
    259, 262–265, 278, 303, 309, 311, 314

General Medical Council, 18, 329
goals, 19, 20, 30–32, 42, 50, 58, 60–62,
    90, 115, 116, 118, 119, 121, 122, 126,
    135, 136, 138, 294, 325–328, 331

hybrid curriculum, 229, 244, 246, 389

imitation, 81
implementation, 9, 57–60, 62–66, 243,
    246
India, 15
Indonesia, 15, 65
initiation, 265
instructional methodology, 4, 6, 7, 69,
    115
internet, 28, 46, 105, 137, 343, 345, 346,
    350
interventional research, 361

Japan, 15
Johnson Wood report, 19

Kirkpatrick, 336, 340
Knowles, 42
Kolb's learning cycle, 35

learner-centered learning, 4, 6, 27–33,
    38, 45, 49, 53, 59, 107, 112, 116, 332,
    345–347, 349, 353
learning objectives, 34, 60–62, 69–71,
    90, 95, 99, 102, 103, 132, 283, 347,
    351, 352
learning objects, 351–353
learning theories, 4, 107, 116, 360
lecture, 6, 14, 17, 18, 21, 30, 32, 36, 37,
    58, 61, 71, 83, 99–103, 105–112, 121,
    124, 131, 347, 352, 361

manipulation, 81, 312
McMaster University, 20, 215, 237, 242
medical education unit, 21, 22, 49, 366,
    367

mentoring, 213
meta-analysis, 363, 364
metacognition, 5, 30, 49–51, 53, 390
microskill, 7
modified essay questions, 237
motivation for learning, 34, 38
multiple choice questions, 297, 361

National University of Singapore, 21,
    359
needs assessment, 349, 391
norm-referenced testing, 185

objective structured clinical
    examination, 320
objectives, 5, 6, 8, 21, 60, 61, 63, 69–71,
    73, 75–78, 85, 86, 89–95, 128, 135,
    136, 287, 297, 326, 329, 331, 338, 339,
    351
objectivity, 283, 284, 293, 303, 309, 313,
    314, 321
observational studies, 364
open-ended questions, 142, 143, 290
oral examination, 8, 309–314

Pakistan, 15
peer teaching, 30, 32, 133
physical examination, 124, 126–128,
    133, 175, 183, 184, 272, 303, 319, 320
portfolio, 8, 37, 325–332
praise, 85
preceptor, 330
probabilistic reasoning, 176
problem-based learning, 6, 20, 30, 38,
    65, 71, 100, 103, 213, 391
psychomotor skills, 133, 392

qualitative studies, 362, 363, 365
quantitative studies, 362
question, 3, 4, 8, 17, 36, 44, 51, 52, 69,
    70, 83–85, 100, 105, 107–112, 117,
    127, 129, 137, 283, 285, 287–291,
    293–306, 312–314, 346, 347, 359, 361,
    363–366, 392
questioning techniques, 137

reflection, 34, 35, 38, 42, 121, 326, 327,
    330, 331, 392
reflective journal entry, 327
reliability, 8, 16, 62, 284, 296, 300–303,
    306, 309–314, 318–321, 329
research, 3, 6, 10, 15, 17, 21–23, 81,
    330–332, 355, 357–367
reviews, 339, 340, 363, 367
role-play, 6, 9, 71, 100, 101, 103,
    131–139

secondary research, 363, 364
self-directed learning, 4, 6, 22, 42, 44,
    50, 53, 325, 328, 332, 345, 346
short answer questions, 303
simulated patients, 318
skills, 3, 5–8, 10, 17, 21, 29–31, 38, 45,
    46, 49, 50, 52, 53, 61, 63, 76–78, 81,
    82, 86, 91, 95, 100–102, 117, 118, 120,
    123, 125, 131, 132, 284, 296, 297, 310,
    311, 319–321, 323, 337, 339, 340, 361
small group, 6, 9, 22, 32, 44, 71, 103,
    115–122, 330, 393
standardized patient, 8, 20, 21, 100,
    318–320, 322, 323
student assessment, 251, 275, 276
summative assessment, 284, 299, 300,
    306, 309–312, 314, 318
surface learning, 32, 33, 38
synthesis, 78, 80, 85, 106, 107, 290, 302,
    306

taxonomy of educational objectives, 86
transfer of learning, 103
trap question, 273, 274
tutor, 32, 62, 117, 118, 121, 122, 138,
    139, 337, 349

validity, 8, 16, 62, 284, 300, 301, 303,
    304, 309, 310, 312–314, 318–320, 329,
    360
verbs
    educational objectives, 5, 21, 71, 73,
        75–78, 85, 86, 89–95, 145,
        195, 231, 258, 276, 287, 297